Reviews of the First Edition of *The Health Care Handbook*

"Two Washington University in St. Louis medical students have written a broad and timely survey of health care in America—equal parts textbook and cheat sheet. Their target audience is fellow med students and those studying in public health and other allied health fields. But *The Health Care Handbook* is a good starting point for any student, health professional, or lay reader interested in how health care is delivered, paid for, researched, supplemented, and debated."

Rob Lott — *Health Affairs*

"This wonderful book by and for students is exactly what it claims to be—a clear and concise guide to the incredibly complex health system we have in the United States. It is chock full of important knowledge; and it is engagingly written. Although the authors invite readers not to read straight through, it is hard to put it down. Initiated by a desire to increase their own understanding of the environment that they were entering as medical students, Elisabeth Askin and Nathan Moore have performed an invaluable service for others."

Stephen C. Schoenbaum, MD, MPH — The Josiah Macy Jr. Foundation

"Medical students Askin and Moore have partnered to write an extremely easy-to-understand book that explains the U.S. health-care system. The book succeeds in making sense of health care without opinion, bias, or dense textbook language. Divided into five chapters, the [first edition] contains a wealth of information that will leave health-care professionals, students, and patients well educated about a system that usually leaves everyone confused."

Booklist

"*The Health Care Handbook* is exactly what it claims to be; "A Clear and Concise Guide to the United States Health Care System." It was researched and written by two medical students who recognized that medical school does not prepare US doctors for dealing with the system in which they practice. The result is one of the best overviews of American health care that I have seen to date."

Thomas W. Byrne — Boston Scientific Corporation

"Written specifically for health professions students, this textbook provides an excellent introduction and overview of the United States health care system. The text offers an illuminating and accessible commentary on a range of key features of this complex system." Dr. Scott Reeves, PhD — UCSF School of Nursing

THE HEALTH CARE HANDBOOK

A Clear and Concise Guide to the United States Health Care System

ELISABETH ASKIN, MD & NATHAN MOORE, MD

SECOND EDITION

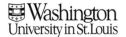
Washington University in St. Louis

SECOND EDITION
First Printing 2014

ISBN 978-0-692-24473-9

Please send questions, comments, and suggestions to: Info@HealthCareHandbook.com
For bulk orders, please visit: HealthCareHandbook.com

Library of Congress Control Number: 2014944562

Funding for this project was provided by the Missouri Foundation for Health, a resource for the region, working with communities and nonprofits to generate and accelerate positive changes in health. As a catalyst for change, the Foundation improves the health of Missourians through partnership, experience, knowledge, and funding.

Editing by Mary Ellen Benson (mebenson26@gmail.com)
Design by John Bennett Graphic Art & Design (JohnBennettGraphics.com)
Fact Checking by Mandy Erickson (MandyErickson.com)

Table of Contents

Foreword

Two years have passed since the publication of the initial version of *The Health Care Handbook*, the pioneering creation of two outstanding Washington University medical students, Elisabeth Askin and Nathan Moore. Strongly motivated by the recognition that many students entering the health professions had little knowledge of the organization, financing, and delivery of health care, they wrote a comprehensive, compact, interesting overview that elicited rave reviews from many individual and institutional experts. The *Handbook* is now in the hands of a large number of students and other interested parties, including health care institutions. A number of medical schools now use the *Handbook* as a foundation for relevant educational programs.

The authors were correct; the *Handbook* satisfies a significant need. They also recognized from the beginning that there must be a second edition. Health care in America is changing significantly, fueled in part by the progressive implementation of the Patient Protection and Affordable Care Act (PPACA). A second edition would include important topics not included in the initial volume and improvements in quality and emphasis in response to very useful feedback from reviewers and readers. The goal is to continue to make the *Handbook* as useful as possible.

Edition Two retains the fundamentals so aptly covered in its predecessor as well as its readable style—replete with appropriate, well-written revisions and new insights that certainly improve its educational value. Updating PPACA presented a special challenge because of the many unforeseen problems associated with the implementation of its major provisions. Given the likelihood of continued downstream uncertainties, the authors have appropriately emphasized the law's key principles and explanations of policy issues in the news associated with the law's rollout. There are timely additions such as a new chapter on quality and technology, a discussion of inter-professional education and teamwork among health professionals, and reviews of specific efforts to improve health care value, for example reducing avoidable hospital readmissions. Another point deserves emphasis. Health care has arguably emerged as the major domestic issue facing all Americans, in part because of its strengths, limitations, and changes. Expanding the health care literacy of students and practitioners in the health professions as well as the lay public is crucial to improving our nation's approach to overall health status. To these ends, Edition Two of *The Health Care Handbook* is an excellent step forward.

On a personal note, Elisabeth's and Nathan's careers have flourished despite the enormous time and effort this book has required. Elisabeth has become a resident in primary care at UCSF and Nathan is now a second-year resident in internal medicine at Barnes-Jewish Hospital. They have already contributed to the health literacy of our profession and are now full-time caregivers. We do attract outstanding young people to the study of medicine.

WILLIAM A. PECK, MD, APRIL 2, 2014

DIRECTOR, CENTER FOR HEALTH POLICY
ALAN A. AND EDITH L. WOLFF DISTINGUISHED PROFESSOR OF MEDICINE
DEAN EMERITUS, WASHINGTON UNIVERSITY SCHOOL OF MEDICINE

Acknowledgments

We received incredible support, commentary, and constructive criticism from our colleagues, family, and friends. First, we'd like to thank William Peck for his mentorship and high expectations. Second, we'd like to thank our significant others, David Askin and Osamuede Osemwota, and our families for all of their love and support. We would also like to thank our fantastic support team: graphic designer John Bennett, editor Mary Ellen Benson, project manager Karen Dodson, grant support Patricia Gregory and Angela Richmond, account managers Amy Meyer and Sarah Kalkbrenner, and problem solver Andrea Sondermann. We completed this edition of the book with the financial backing of the Missouri Foundation for Health, for which we are extremely grateful.

The Washington University School of Medicine community has supported this project from day one. We would like to thank Tom DeFer, Ed Dodson, Gregory Polites, Barbara Sapienza, Alison Whelan, and David Windus for their help. Finally, we have been honored and grateful to receive such backing and interest from the dean of the School of Medicine, Larry Shapiro.

We received invaluable feeback and advice from Jay Albertina, American College of Physician Executives, Peter Angood, Rebekah Apple, Carol Aschenbrener, Aaron Baird, Ryan Barker, Amit Berry, Robert Blaine, Martin Boyer, Janet Brown, Martin Burns, Tom Byrne, Chris Carpenter, LeAnn Chilton, James Christina, Geoff Cislo, Meagan Colvin, John Corker, Kasey Davis, Liz Davlantes, Jennifer Della'Zanna, Susan Deusinger, Rebecca Dresser, Wendy Duncan, Laura Ferguson, Chris Fetter, Andy Flemings, Denise Fletcher, Jess Geeverghese, Lisa Hadley, Kindah Jaradeh, Harry Jonas, Elaine Khoong, Ken King, Napoleon Knight, Cathy Koeln, Ramin Lalezari, Ken Lawson, Josh Levine, Luci Leykum, Steve Lipstein, Rick Majzun, Leonard Marquez, Vicki Martinka, Rebecca McAlister, Phil McGuinness, Jamie Meltzner, Gloria Meredith, Angela Mihalic, Lori Mihalich-Levin, Richard Mahoney, Heidi Miller, Matt Mintz, David Moore, Andrew Morris-Singer, Darilyn Moyer, Harold Mueller,

Phil Needleman, Ryan Nunley, Melissa Palchak, Andrew Pierce, JD Polk, Patricia Potter, Louise Probst, David Pryor, Carl Saubert, Steve Schoenbaum, Alan Schwartz, Matt Shick, Mort Smith, Steve Taff, Mary Taylor, Victor Trogdon, Judy VandeWater, Ed Weisbart, Michael Weiss, Mary White, Sue Wintz, Amy Yu, and Kevin Zeng.

We would further like to give thanks to all of the professors and staff at Washington University School of Medicine for creating an atmosphere of such encouragement, assistance, and belief in students' potential.

Introduction

Why We Wrote This Book

When we were first getting interested in health care, a few years before starting medical school, we tried to cobble together an understanding of what health care even was. We found ourselves lost in a sea of confusion, faced with highly specialized publications that were often ideologically bent. Sure, generalized textbooks are out there, but even those seemed to focus on policy without explaining the huge world of research and drug companies that we kept reading about in the news. Besides, let's face it: Textbooks are boring. Even a motivated student can only read so much from textbooks without being required to.

In writing this book, we've worked hard to rid our knowledge base of huge gaps, vague opinions, and biased perceptions of some issues. But it shouldn't be so hard, especially not for health professions students, and especially not in a nation where health care is such a huge, important, costly industry. We should make it as easy as possible to understand the U.S. health care system.

Once we published the book, we tried to get as much feedback as possible—from students, from patients, from providers, from academics, from industry experts. This second edition has incorporated their feedback.

OUR GOALS

The goal of this book is to provide a broad base of facts, concepts, and analysis so the reader gets a thorough overview of the American health care system. The goal is to be exhaustive in breadth rather than in depth, to make sure the reader never gets into an argument about health care only to have his or her opponent bring up a completely unfamiliar issue, to provide a baseline level of facts and analysis so that readers may go forth with the ability not only to understand and evaluate what they read but also to form their own opinions.

At the same time, the goal is to balance accurate, nuanced, up-to-date content with a compact, readable format. Since nuance and brevity don't usually go hand in hand, at times we have had to make concessions on one side or the other.

Finally, a goal of this book is to impress a single theme upon the reader: **Everything is always more complicated than you think.** (If we could have underlined that phrase obsessively in each copy of this book, we would have.) It's frustrating to know so much yet know so little; to think there's a solution if only it weren't thwarted by reality. But understanding these complications is necessary not only for understanding health care but also for developing informed, nuanced, realistic opinions. It would have been obnoxious to put this disclaimer on every page of the book, so we'll just ask you to keep it in mind as you read: *It's more complicated than this!*

INTENDED AUDIENCE

Because we're students ourselves, we have firsthand insight into what students don't know, what they want to know, and what they need to know. As such, students are our primary focus. On the other hand, we wanted to learn these things *before* we were students. Certainly these topics are relevant to all who have an interest in health care, public policy, or how our government spends money. And aren't we all students of what we want to learn? Thus, our focus is on "students" in the broad sense of the word.

A lot of people from different walks of life have read this book—from the CEO of a major hospital to experts whose research we cited to journalists to fellow students to our moms—and we have used their feedback to make the book as useful as possible to as many people as possible. That said, it's not quite feasible to set out to write a book for "everybody." We think the book will hold the most value for the following:

> ▶ **Students** in undergraduate, graduate, and professional programs focused on medicine, nursing, dentistry, pharmacy, allied health, medical research, biotechnology, public health, public policy,

economics, finance, health care administration, business, and law. Heck, throw in history and political science, too!

▸ **Health care professionals** who want to expand their knowledge about what affects them in the workplace or who want a reference for continuing education.

▸ **Lay readers** who are sufficiently interested in learning more about health care to have started reading a book about it. In short, if you ever find yourself confused by a news article about what an Accountable Care Organization is, or you don't have quite enough information to argue with your Uncle Dan about pharmaceutical companies, or you're annoyed that everything you read has an agenda—then this book is for you.

LIMITATIONS

This book can't cover everything, and it's not for everyone. We decided not to include certain topics, and those we did include have depths we didn't plumb. If someone, for instance, has been working in health administration for the past 25 years, he or she will think this book misses some important nuances.

Well, that reader would be right, which is the point. Our book is a survey, not a deep dive. We've tried to address this limitation by pointing to **suggested** reading and reminding you of how complicated the issues are. However, if you're looking for an in-depth nuanced exploration of limited topics, this isn't the right book for you.

HOW TO READ THE BOOK

First, as we said previously, we don't want this to be a boring textbook. While the book is ordered as a progression of knowledge, it isn't necessary to read straight through, **cover to cover**. Rather, the book is separated into distinct sections, which you can flip around and/or read selectively to supplement knowledge you already have. (Though we should mention that Chapter 5 on Policy and Reform is harder to fully understand without the first four chapters if you don't already have background knowledge in health care.) See the extensive Table of Contents to get an idea of the sections and what you might want to peruse.

Second, we've done our best to identify useful resources for the interested reader. See the "Suggested Reading" section on page 224 and at HealthCareHandbook.com/SuggestedReading. Further, you'll find cross-references in parentheses that point to other relevant sections.

Third, you should read keeping the golden triad of health care Cost-Access-Quality (see next page) always in mind. Pretty much any information, problem, or solution falls into Cost, Access, and/or Quality; the three are an interdependent cycle rather than separate pillars. We'll refer to the triad at various points, and, even when we don't—even when you're just musing on the issues—you should wonder how not just one but all may be affected.

Finally, we want to hear from you! Please visit HealthCareHandbook.com to see the latest news on the book, and send all questions, comments, and suggestions to Info@HealthCareHandbook.com. We'll read each and every last email because we truly want your feedback.

ELISABETH ASKIN AND NATHAN MOORE, SEPTEMBER 2014

Before You Begin:
Understanding the Lay of the Land

Before we dive in to the *Handbook,* let's take a minute to give you the state of the U.S. health care system today by using the standard Cost-Access-Quality framework to analyze health systems.

Cost

The U.S. currently spends more than 17% of its national gross domestic product (GDP) on health care, far more than any other country in the world. Health care spending now averages almost $9,000 per American,[1] and health care is the fastest growing industry in the country.[2] Private (nongovernmental) health care spending accounts for a large portion of the difference between spending in the U.S. and in other industrialized countries.

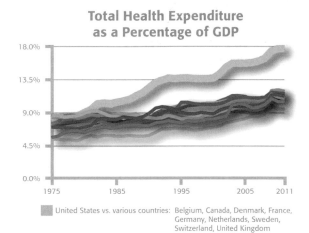

Total Health Expenditure as a Percentage of GDP

United States vs. various countries: Belgium, Canada, Denmark, France, Germany, Netherlands, Sweden, Switzerland, United Kingdom

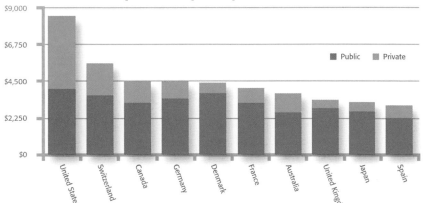

Health Expenditure per Capita 2011 (or Nearest Year)

Public   Private

United States, Switzerland, Canada, Germany, Denmark, France, Australia, United Kingdom, Japan, Spain

(top and bottom) ***Organisation for Economic Co-operation and Development, "Health Statistics 2013," June 2013.*** *Note: Values in U.S. $ Purchasing Power Parity. Data for Japan and Australia refers to 2008.*

Access

The U.S. has fewer physicians, hospital beds, physician visits, and hospitalizations per capita than most other industrialized countries.[3] Eighty-five percent of Americans report having a regular source of ongoing care, but more than a quarter encounter difficulty accessing the health care system.[4] There are large disparities in access by type of health insurance coverage.

People who Were Unable to Get or Delayed in Getting Needed Medical Care, Dental Care, or Prescription Medicines in the Last 12 Months

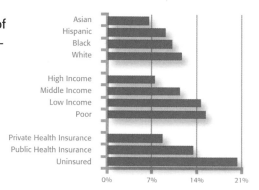

Agency for Healthcare Research and Quality, "2012 National Healthcare Quality and Disparities Reports," June 2013. Note: Health insurance status refers to those 18–64 years old. Poor refers to household incomes below the federal poverty level (FPL); low income, 100–200% FPL; middle, 200–399% FPL; high, more than 400% FPL.

Access to Doctor or Nurse When Sick or Need Care

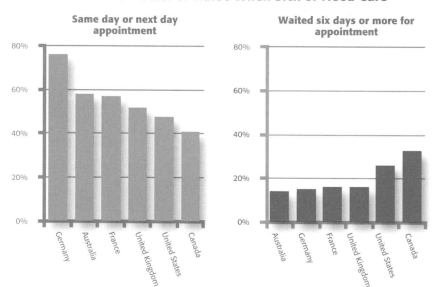

The Commonwealth Fund, "2013 International Health Policy Survey in Eleven Countries," Nov. 2013. Used with permission.

Quality

Despite spending all that money, we don't have the highest quality health system. Americans only receive about 55–70% of recommended care they need,[4,5] and huge disparities exist in health outcomes by insurance status, race, income, and location.[6] Life expectancy is rising, but not as fast as in other industrialized countries. The U.S. ranks poorly for infant and maternal mortality, preventive care, and chronic disease care. On the bright side, we're near the front of the pack in cancer care, medical research and education, and diagnostic imaging.[3]

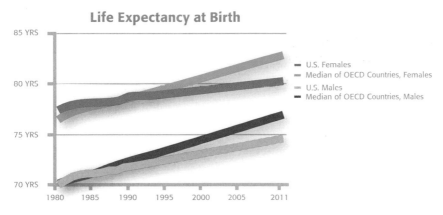

Organisation for Economic Co-operation and Development,
"Health Statistics 2013," June 2013.

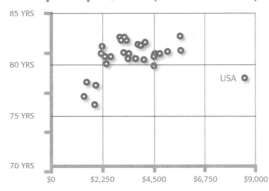

Organisation for Economic Co-operation and Development,
"Health Statistics 2013," June 2013.

Potential Years of Life Lost

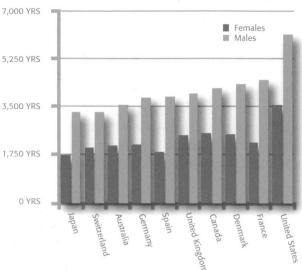

Organisation for Economic Co-operation and Development, "Health Statistics 2011," June 2011. Note: Data from 2009, or nearest year.

Any way you slice it, the U.S. health care system is in trouble. The most recent major international comparison by the Commonwealth Fund ranked our system 7th—which isn't so bad until you realize that the study only included seven countries.

Overall Ranking (2010)

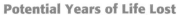

	AUS	CAN	GER	NETH	NZ	UK	US
Overall Ranking (2010)	3	6	4	1	5	2	7
Quality Care	4	7	5	2	1	3	6
Effective Care	2	7	6	3	5	1	4
Safe Care	6	5	3	1	4	2	7
Coordinated Care	4	5	7	2	1	3	6
Patient-Centered Care	2	5	3	6	1	7	4
Access	6.5	5	3	1	4	2	6.5
Cost-Related Problem	6	3.5	3.5	2	5	1	7
Timeliness of Care	6	7	2	1	3	4	5
Efficiency	2	6	5	3	4	1	7
Equity	4	5	3	1	6	2	7
Long, Healthy, Productive Lives	1	2	3	4	5	6	7
Health Expenditures/Capita	$3,586	$4,184	$4,272	$4,656	$3,020	$3,064	$7,919

Adapted from Davis, et al., "Mirror, Mirror on the Wall: How the Performance of the U.S. Health Care System Compares Internationally–2010 Update," The Commonwealth Fund, June 2010. Used with permission.

To quote from an amazing 2013 article in JAMA called "The Anatomy of Health Care in the United States":[2]

> *"The breadth and consistency of the U.S. under performance across disease categories suggests that the United States pays a penalty for its extreme fragmentation, financial incentives that favor procedures over comprehensive longitudinal care, and absence of organizational strategy at the individual system level."*

References

1. NHE Fact Sheet. www.cms.gov/Research-Statistics-Data-and-Systems/Statistics-Trends-and-Reports/NationalHealthExpendData/NHE-Fact-Sheet.html. Accessed July 8, 2014.
2. Moses H, Matheson D, et al. The Anatomy of Health Care in the United States. *JAMA: The Journal of the American Medical Association.* 2013;310(18):1947-1964.
3. David S. The U.S. Health System in Perspective: A Comparison of Twelve Industrialized Nations. www.commonwealthfund.org/~/media/Files/Publications/Issue%20Brief/2011/Jul/1532_Squires_US_hlt_sys_comparison_12_nations_intl_brief_v2.pdf. Accessed July 21, 2014.
4. AHRQ. 2012 National Healthcare Quality Report. www.ahrq.gov/research/findings/nhqrdr/nhqr12. Accessed July 21, 2014.
5. Asch SM, Kerr EA, et al. Who Is at Greatest Risk for Receiving Poor-Quality Health Care? *New England Journal of Medicine.* 2006;354(11):1147-1156.
6. AHRQ. 2012 National Healthcare Disparities Report. nhqrnet.ahrq.gov/inhqrdr/reports/nhdr. Accessed July 21, 2014.

Chapter 1
Health Care Systems and Delivery

Let's say your watch is running slow. You know the time is wrong, but, chances are, you don't know how to fix it. Instead, you take it to the watchmaker, who understands the inner workings of the gears and how their interaction produces that time, right or wrong. To truly understand the function, you must understand the mechanism. It's time to think like a watchmaker. To make better sense of the U.S. health care system, let's get started by examining all of the parts and how they work together. Then we'll discuss some of the issues facing that system today.

HEALTH CARE SYSTEMS can be categorized in many different ways. We'll start with the two broadest categories—inpatient vs. outpatient care—and whittle down from there. First, let's define these terms:

Inpatient: Traditionally, this was a patient who got admitted to a medical facility for at least one night—but now it's not so simple (see, things got complicated from the first page![a]). These medical facilities are hospitals, mental institutions, and nursing homes.
Outpatient: Patient is examined, diagnosed, or treated at a medical facility but doesn't stay overnight.

The distinction can be tricky, though, because inpatient facilities—e.g., hospitals—usually have outpatient centers in them. So you don't have to be an inpatient to be treated at a hospital. This intersection reflects the complexity of medical categories in general. They often blur, overlap, and mix together.

Hospitals

Focusing on hospitals, let's examine the types of administration, types of services, organization, and operations.

Breakdown of 5,634 U.S. Hospitals

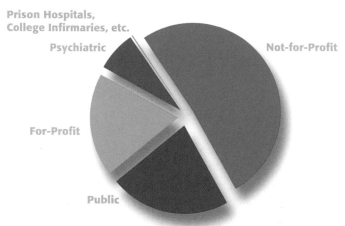

Prison Hospitals, College Infirmaries, etc.

Psychiatric

Not-for-Profit

For-Profit

Public

American Hospital Association, "Fast Facts on US Hospitals," Jan. 2014. Used with permission. *Note: This does not include long-term care hospitals.*

---

a   Patients can be in "observation" in the emergency department for more than 24 hours. As of October 2013, Medicare defines an "inpatient" as someone who stays in the hospital for at least two midnights.

Ownership

Public: Operated either by the federal, state, or local government.

▸ **Federal:** Three federal government agencies operate hospitals—the Department of Defense for active military members, the Indian Health Service for Native Americans, and the Veterans Health Administration for military veterans.

  ▸ **VA:** The Department of Veterans Affairs (VA) operates 152 hospitals and 821 outpatient clinics nationwide.[1] Note three interesting things about VA hospitals: First, their patients are more likely to be elderly and male than the general population. Second, the VA was an early adopter of electronic medical records in the mid-to-late 1990s. Third, while a number of studies have shown the VA to have excellent quality in chronic disease and preventive care,[2] the system is still sometimes plagued by scandals over poor quality care.

▸ **State/Local** (i.e., "public"): State hospitals are typically long-term facilities for psychiatric patients. Most public hospitals, though, are safety-net, general hospitals that maintain a primary focus on free or reduced-cost care for underserved populations. In 2012, there were 1,037 state and local hospitals.[3]

▸ **Prisons:** Prison hospitals are administered by federal, state, or local governments, or by private contractors.

Private: Hospitals not operated by the government. However, note that all hospitals that accept Medicare and Medicaid are, in some sense, *funded* by the government.

▸ **Not-for-Profit:** Not-for-profit institutions, particularly religious ones, are hospital mainstays that historically stem from charity institutions for the poor. Profit is reinvested in the hospital or community, rather than given to shareholders. These hospitals typically maintain a commitment to charity care, though this is often not their primary focus. Some not-for-profit hospitals function as safety-net hospitals; recognizing the community benefit of the charity care they provide, the government doesn't require these hospitals to pay taxes.[b,4]

  ▸ **Secular:** Most not-for-profit hospitals are owned and operated

---

b   Though we should note the difference between a "not-for-profit" and a "charity care" hospital. They overlap but are not the same.

by non-religious civic organizations. They are governed by a board of directors composed of locally prominent citizens.

> **Religious:** Many religious organizations have opened hospitals over the years, seeking to serve their own population, the underserved, or the community at large. Religious hospitals make up 14% of all hospitals in the U.S., and most of these are Catholic.[5] The direct impact of the religious organization on the day-to-day management of the hospital varies; in one arrangement, religious leaders comprise a portion of the board of directors but a lay CEO operates the hospital.

> **For-Profit:** For-profit hospitals are owned by private corporations and some of the hospital's profit is given to shareholders (as opposed to all of it being reinvested into operations). Unlike not-for-profit hospitals, these organizations are required to pay taxes.[c] The largest operator of for-profit hospitals is the Hospital Corporation of America, which owns and operates 165 hospitals across the country.[6]

> **Physician-Owned Hospitals:** As of 2013, the U.S. had over 260 physician-owned hospitals.[7] The majority are for-profit institutions. These hospitals can be of any type but are more likely to be single-specialty—especially orthopedics, oncology, or cardiology—than hospitals that don't have physician owners.[8] The Affordable Care Act included new restrictions on expansion of physician-owned hospitals (see Chapter 5 for more).

Services

Another way to classify hospitals is by services offered. Note that any of these types of hospitals may be associated with any sort of ownership.

General: Even aside from the soap opera, general hospitals are the most well-known types. They supply a range of services, including emergency services, OB/GYN, internal medicine, surgery, and a variety of others.

> **Teaching:** The U.S. has nearly 400 major teaching hospitals.[9] They're connected with medical schools, have residency programs, and are often referred to as "academic medical centers." Teaching hospitals explicitly include the training of medical students, residents, and other health care professionals as part of their mission. They're

---

c   These hospitals also by law must provide emergency room care (that is, enough care to "stabilize" a patient) regardless of ability to pay, in effect providing some charity care.

usually large hospitals located in major urban centers and provide a significant amount of charity care.

Specialty: Some hospitals—or sections of general hospitals—focus solely on a single specialty, such as cardiology, oncology, or women's medicine. Children's and psychiatric hospitals fall into this category as well.

▸ **Children's:** These may be general hospitals for children, or they may be a section of a medical–surgical hospital. There are about 250 of these[10] in the U.S., many of which also serve as teaching and research institutions.

▸ **Psychiatric:** The U.S. has 413 of these institutions.[3] All focus solely on mental disorders, although they vary widely in breadth of services and in size. Psychiatric hospitals may treat mainly outpatients or short-term inpatients, or they may focus on long-term care.

Networks

Most hospitals are part of a health care delivery system or network,[3] an organization that owns and operates multiple hospitals and/or outpatient facilities.

▸ **Horizontal Network:** This is a conglomeration of multiple institutions of the same type. An example is Shriners Hospitals, which owns and operates 22 pediatric hospitals across the country.[11]

▸ **Vertical Network:** This contains different types of services. An example is Kaiser Permanente, a network of organizations that function variously as an insurer, an owner of hospitals and outpatient centers, and an employer of physicians.

Please note that many organizations of health care providers are also called networks. Those are detailed in Chapter 3.

Organization

In 2012, U.S. hospitals had a combined total of a million beds, 37 million admissions, and $829 *billion* in expenses.[3] This means a hospital is a big business, and operating one is just as complex, if not more so, than operating any other large corporation. Far more services—and people—make the hospital run than any patient will ever encounter:

▸ **Board of Directors/Trustees:** This small group sets the strategic vision for the hospital, provides oversight of the hospital's finances and quality, and hires and fires the CEO. Directors are typically paid at for-profit institutions and serve without compensation at not-for-profit hospitals.

▸ **Administrative Services:** These workers—the CEO, vice presidents, department heads, etc.—run the hospital on a day-to-day basis. They execute hospital policy, manage finances and budgetary planning, and handle marketing and public relations.

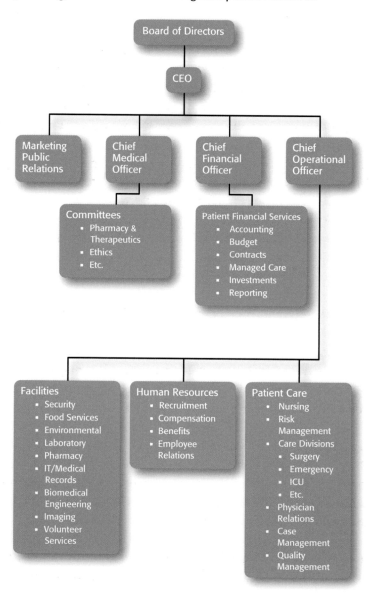

> **Therapeutic Services:** These workers provide the care normally associated with hospitals, such as physician visits, drugs, surgery, physical therapy, social work, psychiatry, etc. These are the services that directly make the patient feel better.

> **Diagnostic Services:** These workers administer the laboratory, testing, and imaging facilities that help those in therapeutic services to figure out what care is needed.

> **Informational Services:** These workers document and process information, such as medical records, billing, admissions, human resources, computer systems, and health education. Some of this may be performed by employees in dedicated roles (e.g., medical billers) and some by other staff (e.g., nurses performing registration).

> **Support Services:** These workers maintain the hospital as a functioning facility. Areas of operation include food services, supply management, maintaining biotechnology equipment, and housekeeping.

> **Committees:** Each hospital has a number of committees, many of which are headed by the medical staff, that make decisions regarding hospital management, regulation, and the care delivered in that institution. A few of these committees include Pharmacy and Therapeutics, Infection Control, and Quality Improvement.

Non-Hospital Inpatient Facilities

Thousands of non-hospital facilities also provide inpatient care.

Skilled Nursing Facilities: (commonly called nursing homes) These provide 24-hour nursing care and assistance with daily living. In 2012, the 15,673 skilled nursing facilities in the U.S. had a total of more than 1.7 million patient beds.[12] Residents include the elderly as well as younger patients with permanent or temporary disabilities. Stays can be as brief as three days, although typically Medicare will cover up to 30 days for rehabilitation. Further, some patients who cannot live independently or be cared for at home will live out their days in a nursing home. Most skilled nursing facilities are privately administered but often receive a large share of their funding through Medicare and Medicaid.

Long-Term Acute Care Hospitals: These serve patients who need intensive, hospital-level care for weeks or months. Patients in these hospitals typically have multiple, complex medical problems. In 2012, there were 420 in the U.S.[13]

Inpatient Rehab Facilities: Also known as Acute Rehabilitation Hospitals, these facilities care for patients who require comprehensive rehabilitation along with medical management. Patients often enter these facilities after strokes, serious fractures, or joint replacement surgeries. In 2012, there were 1,166 in the U.S.[13]

The above three types of facilities—together termed "post-acute care"— have experienced rapid growth in the past 20 years and are an increasing area of concern for Medicare spending and quality improvement.

Outpatient Care

Outpatient care is often referred to as "ambulatory" care, the idea being that you can walk in (and hopefully out) on your own. However, the strict definition of an outpatient is a person receiving medical care without staying overnight at a health care facility. Outpatient visits may include minor surgery, check-ups, physical therapy, mammograms, and lab testing, to name a few examples.

That variety in care is reflected in this section, as we look at some of the types of facilities, services, and organizations common in outpatient care, keeping in mind that these may mix and match.

Outpatient Visits to Physicians in 2010[12]
81% to Physicians' Offices
▸ 55% Primary Care / 45% Specialist
8% to Hospital-Based Outpatient Services
10% to the Emergency Department

Delivery Formats for Outpatient Medicine

Private Practice: An outpatient clinic owned and operated by the health care professionals who practice there. Private practice has traditionally been the dominant form of outpatient care in the U.S. (though this model is dying out). Private practices are often classified in two ways: solo or group, and physician-owned or physician-employed.

Hospital/Health Care Network: As discussed in "The Hospital–Physician

Relationship" section of this chapter, an increasing number of physicians are employed directly by hospitals or health care networks. In many cases, a private group practice will be purchased by a hospital or health care network. These physicians, now employees, may be integrated into normal hospital operations, be housed in a separate section of the building, or practice in traditional community-based locations.

Community Health Center (CHC): These are government-supported clinics that provide low-cost care to underserved and low-income populations. CHCs often focus on primary care but may offer a range of services in a "one-stop shop" format. For instance, some CHCs offer laboratory testing, OB/GYN, behavioral health, and dental services in addition to primary care. In 2014, more than 9,000 CHCs were providing care to 22 million patients annually.[14] Many CHCs are also designated as Federally Qualified Health Centers, which enables them to receive extra funding from Medicare, Medicaid, and CHIP. FQHCs are slated to receive expanded funding under the ACA.

Free/Charitable Clinic: These clinics also offer care for underserved and low-income populations, but are funded and operated by private not-for-profit organizations.

Local Government: Apart from funding other institutions, many city and county health departments directly offer a limited range of outpatient services, including immunizations and screening for diseases such as tuberculosis and HIV.[15]

Emergency Department (ED): Care received in the ED is considered outpatient care because those patients have not yet been admitted to the inpatient section of the hospital. There is a big demand for emergency medicine physicians, and many EDs, especially those in rural areas, end up being staffed by physicians who have completed residencies in fields other than emergency medicine.

Urgent Care Center (UCC): UCCs bridge the gap between primary care and the ED. They're open on evenings and weekends, appealing to patients who can't get same-day appointments with their primary care physicians, need medical care outside of normal office hours, or don't have regular primary care physicians. However, UCCs aren't equipped to deal with trauma or true medical emergencies. UCCs are primarily staffed by physicians trained in family medicine, nurse practitioners and physician assistants, and about half of all centers are physician-owned. The most common services offered by UCCs are laceration and fracture care, X-rays, school and employment physicals, and immunizations.[16] There are approximately 9,000 UCCs with each center seeing an average of 342 patients per week.[17]

Retail Clinic: These small medical clinics in convenient locations (e.g., Walgreens) offer quick, inexpensive, protocol-based care for limited medical conditions, such as strep throat, minor burns, and vaccinations. Patients who present with urgent or more complicated conditions are referred to EDs, UCCs, or other local physicians. Most retail clinics are staffed by nurse practitioners, although some employ physician assistants and physicians. The number of retail clinics nationwide has grown from 200 in 2006 to 1,649 in 2014.[18]

Ambulatory Surgery Center (ASC): Although surgical services are often closely linked with hospitals, more than 60% of surgical procedures in the U.S. are actually performed in outpatient settings.[12] ASCs are like surgical clinics, where patients can undergo minor surgical procedures that don't require hospital stays. The most common procedures performed at the 5,260 ASCs[19] in the U.S. are colonoscopies, endoscopies, and cataract removals.[20] More than 80% of ASCs are owned at least in part by physicians, which can create conflict of interest. For instance, studies indicate that physician-owners of ASCs are more likely to recommend surgery for their patients than are other physicians.[21]

Home Care: About 12 million Americans receive health care in their homes[22] rather than traveling to health care institutions. Many patients are discharged from hospitals while needing long-term treatment and oversight, which can be accomplished for less cost in the home than in an inpatient facility. The primary professionals who provide home care are home health aides and nurses. The primary caregivers, though, are non-professional family members. Estimates indicate that 65 million Americans care for loved ones in the home with chronic conditions, disabilities, disease, or the frailties of old age.[23] The "average" U.S. caregiver is a 49-year-old woman who works outside the home and spends nearly 20 hours per week providing unpaid care to her mother for nearly five years.[24] At-home care is likely to get emphasized more as the U.S. population ages and health care reimbursement models change.

Hospice: These programs shift emphasis to maximize quality of life rather than "quantity" of life for patients with terminal illnesses. Care is focused on providing comfort from their symptoms, including pain control, rather than attempting to cure. More than 40% of the people who died in 2011 were under the care of a hospice program at the time of death.[25] Hospice care is less expensive than typical inpatient care, and, interestingly, patients in hospice care may live longer than those who continue medical treatment.[26]

Non-Physician Services: Dentists, chiropractors, podiatrists, physical therapists, and optometrists are just a few of the providers who practice primarily in outpatient settings. Modern medicine increasingly recognizes the value of multidisciplinary clinical teams. See Chapter 6 for more about different types of health care providers and how they work together.

Complementary and Alternative Medicine: More than one-third of Americans regularly use complementary (used with conventional medicine) or alternative (used in place of conventional medicine) therapies, which include herbal or natural products, acupuncture, and homeopathic care. Most complementary and alternative medicine (CAM) is provided in an outpatient setting. Although some insurance plans provide reimbursement for CAM services, the majority of spending is out of pocket and totals more than $30 billion annually.[27] Upon hearing the rate of use and spending on CAM, it's not surprising that the federal government has established a National Center for CAM to study the field.

Patient-Centered Medical Home: This model is for comprehensive and coordinated outpatient care. For more information, see page 17.

Boutique/Concierge Practice: These clinics focus on patients who would like a high level of service (e.g., short wait times, long appointments, and physicians who are available 24/7) and are willing to pay for it. Boutique or concierge practices typically charge an annual membership fee, sometimes along with separate appointment fees, and can therefore afford to keep the total patient load low and have more time for each patient. Note, however, that these patients still would want insurance for any care not provided in the office.

Issues in Health Care Delivery

Primary Care Crisis

The percentage of U.S. physicians working in primary care has been on the decline for some time, and today fewer than 40% of practicing physicians are in primary care.[28] In 2010, there were 209,000 primary care physicians and 86,000 primary care nurse practitioners and physician assistants.[29] A large workload falls on these providers' shoulders. Duke University researchers estimate that, given the typical patient load and the current guidelines for care, a PCP should be spending 7.4 hours per day on preventive care,[30] 10.6 hours on managing chronic diseases,[31] and 4.6 hours on handling acute illness[32]—totaling 22.6 hours a day.[d]

Generalists and Specialists as a Share of all Doctors

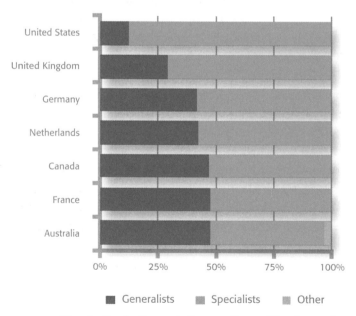

Generalists ■ Specialists ■ Other

Organisation for Economic Co-operation and Development, "Health at a Glance 2013," Nov. 2013. Note: Generalists include general practitioners/ family doctors and other generalist (non-specialist) medical practitioners. Specialists include pediatricians, obstetricians/gynecologists, psychiatrists, medical, surgical and other specialists. Other includes medical doctors not further defined.

---

d   Which is certainly not feasible—only residents work that many hours a day!

This trend has many causes: higher pay for specialists than for primary care physicians (PCPs), the low status of primary care in most academic medical centers, and unpleasant workloads (too much paperwork, too many patients per day). Compounding the problem, over the years, hundreds of primary care residency slots have been cut or converted to specialty training positions,[33] decreasing the number of new PCPs. Not surprisingly, this has led to a shortage of primary care providers throughout the country. The federal government estimates that 60 million Americans live in primary care shortage areas,[34] a number that has continued to increase in recent years.

So, why should we care? What's so bad about fewer primary care physicians and more specialists? Everyone seems to want to see a specialist, anyway! To answer, let's look at the issues of cost, access, and quality.

Cost: In 2005, a systematic review of research about primary care usage and health outcomes found that "areas with higher ratios of primary care physicians to population had much lower total health care costs than did other areas, possibly partly because of better preventive care and lower hospitalization rates. [. . .] In contrast, [greater] supply of specialists was associated with more spending and poorer care."[35]

Access: Primary care is the easiest way for most people to access health services, both for ongoing wellness or disease management and for appropriate referrals to specialists.

Quality: Use of primary care leads to better health outcomes.[e] The same systematic review noted above found that primary care was associated with better outcomes in all-cause mortality, heart disease mortality, stroke mortality, infant mortality, low birth weight, life expectancy, and self-rated health.[35]

Primary care creates this benefit through six mechanisms:
  ▸ Greater access to needed services
  ▸ Better quality of care
  ▸ A greater focus on prevention
  ▸ Early management of health problems
  ▸ The cumulative effect of the main primary care delivery characteristics

---

e   Note that, while the evidence shows this to be true on the population level, individual patients with specific conditions do better with specialty care. It's still good to send heart failure patients to see a cardiologist.

▶ The role of primary care in reducing unnecessary and potentially harmful specialist care[35]

This list shows that a shortage of primary care providers may lead to poor quality, high costs, and restricted access. The Affordable Care Act may only exacerbate this problem—over the next decade, millions of newly insured Americans will be looking for primary care providers. They may be in for a rude surprise when they find that many primary care providers won't take new patients with Medicaid or Medicare; of those who do, the wait for an appointment may be one month or more.[36]

So how can we fix the problem of a primary care provider shortage in the U.S.? Here are some potential solutions, although each has pros and cons:

▶ Reduce medical education debt.
▶ Tweak current payment systems (like Relative Value Units, page 50) to increase reimbursement for primary care services.
▶ Use alternate payment systems that reward health promotion and coordination of care rather than costly procedures. Physicians point to the fact that diagnosis comes primarily from history-taking, yet interviewing a patient is poorly reimbursed.
▶ Reduce the hassles of primary care practice (e.g., less paperwork, longer patient visits, etc.).
▶ Increase the number of residency positions in primary care training programs.
▶ Expand the role of non-physician providers, like physician assistants and nurse practitioners, in the primary care team.
▶ Expand the Patient-Centered Medical Home and other delivery structures that put the PCP in charge of coordinating patient care across medical specialties.
▶ Establish more three-year medical schools—cheaper and faster— aimed at producing family physicians. One program already doing this is the Texas Tech Family Medicine Accelerated Track.

Changing Models of Care

In the 20th century, health care benefited from a revolution of technological and pharmacological advances. In the 21st century, the revolution will be in how care is delivered. Expect big changes.

CHANGING PRACTICE PATTERNS

For physicians who work primarily in outpatient settings, the dominant trend over the last 30 years has been a shift from working in solo private practices to group practices. In fact, the proportion of physicians in solo practice has declined by more than 40% during this time period[37,38] —30% just since 2000[39]—and a growing number of physician practices are now owned by hospitals or health care networks.[f] This represents a fundamental change for physicians.

Why is this change occurring? Although the outpatient practices of physician employees, especially in primary care, may be unprofitable for the network,[39] money is made when patients are referred to specialists, sent for lab testing and imaging, or admitted to the hospital. Also, new payment systems that reward comprehensive services, coordination of care, and risk reduction favor large networks that can provide primary, inpatient, and specialist care, such as Accountable Care Organizations. From the physician's perspective, being an employee doesn't look so bad when it means your practice doesn't have to foot the bill for a new electronic health record, the implementation of government regulations, malpractice insurance, or administrative overhead.

However, being an employee means that doctors can sometimes butt heads with hospital administration. Though both medical and administrative staff wants what is best for patient care, they may emphasize different aspects of what that means. Most salient is when what health care staff considers good medicine is what administrators consider a poor allocation of resources (and, as administrators would point out, "poor allocation" for one patient may lead to fewer resources to properly care for other patients, which is bad medicine). For the most part, these goals align, but at times they diverge, and power struggles may arise.[40]

One potential area of disagreement is the purchasing of equipment and prioritizing what treatments are offered. For instance, an increasing number of prostate surgeries are performed with high-tech robotic equipment; these systems cost upwards of a million dollars each. When considering

---

f   Some physicians are directly employed by insurance companies rather than hospitals or health care networks. This arrangement is discussed in Chapter 2.

whether to purchase one, the surgeon (who uses the equipment) and administrator (who pays for it) are likely to ask different questions:

Surgeon	Administrator
▸ Will this improve my patients' outcomes?	▸ Will this improve patients' outcomes?
▸ Will this make surgeries easier and/or quicker for me?	▸ Is the system a good value? Could this same amount of money be spent elsewhere in the hospital and help more patients?
▸ What's the learning curve for the new instrument? Will the hospital staff be properly trained?	▸ Will insurance companies reimburse more now to compensate for our increased costs?
▸ Will I lose patients if I don't have this system?	▸ Will I lose physicians if I don't have this system?
▸ Is this product coming from my preferred vendor?	▸ Will the hospital save money if all surgeons use a product from the same vendor?

So, how will this dramatic change in the hospital–physician relationship affect patients? A variety of outcomes are possible. In the best case scenario, the integration of primary care and specialist physicians with hospital administration will foster greater coordination between providers, fewer duplicated labs and procedures, and more efficient delivery of care, leading to better outcomes and lower costs for patients. In the worst case, decreased market competition due to dominance of a few large, integrated hospital–physician networks could lead to poorer outcomes and higher costs for patients. The true result will likely fall somewhere in between, but expect the changing nature of the hospital–physician relationship to remain an important and controversial issue.

TRENDING FROM OUTPATIENT TO INPATIENT TO OUTPATIENT

In the olden days, physicians usually made home visits, or house calls, so the majority of patients were by definition outpatients. With the advent of antiseptic facilities and surgery, hospitals ceased to be places where sick people went to die and started to be places where sick people went to get well. So the 20th century saw the rise of the inpatient.

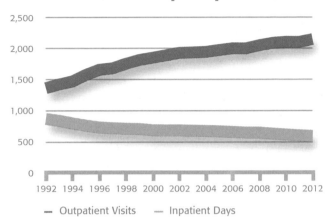

Community Hospitals: Inpatient vs. Outpatient Utilization per Capita

— Outpatient Visits   — Inpatient Days

American Hospital Association, "TrendWatch Chartbook," March 2014.
Used with permission. Note: Data per 1,000 persons.

However, over the past 20 years, the balance has again shifted and outpatient care represents an increasing share of dollars and attention. Today, outpatient care accounts for about 40% of health care spending,[41] but, as you can see from the figure above, outpatient care accounts for a much greater proportion of hospital visits.

Two other trends are bringing care way out of the hospital; home visits—a return to how doctors used to practice—and telemedicine, a new way of practicing, allowing doctors to "see" patients in remote areas.

PATIENT-CENTERED MEDICAL HOMES

A Patient-Centered Medical Home (PCMH) is a new model of delivering and financing health care by creating a single center through which all of a patient's care is coordinated, with bundled payments. The idea is that all-inclusive care can be more efficient and of better quality.

It is rooted in primary care with several goals:[42]

▸ **Comprehensive, team-based care:** Recognition that care doesn't begin and end with a physician. The PCMH includes nurse practitioners, nurses, medical assistants, pharmacists, social workers, nutritionists, health educators, and sometimes mental health and laboratory services.

17

- ▶ **Coordinated care:** The PCMH tracks records and follows patients through their "transitions" (see Chapter 3) to specialists and inpatient admissions, or any other care the patient may receive.
- ▶ **Improved quality and safety:** Using evidence (research) to design the best delivery of care, and then tracking outcomes. One important element is the use of health IT such as a comprehensive electronic medical record and electronic prescribing.
- ▶ **Improved access:** Patients should be able to make appointments quickly (often same-day or within a few days), as well as to access providers over the phone or email when they need to.

PCMHs may be financed through private insurance, state government (through Medicaid/CHIP), or the federal government (i.e., the VA or Medicare).[43] Reimbursements may be structured along several lines, most importantly involving bundled payments; i.e., a fixed amount paid per patient per month to cover all actions the PCMH may make during that time. The goal with such payment (quite different from most models of financing care, see Chapter 2) is to incentivize more efficient care. However, the PCMH may also receive payments based on the more traditional fee-for-service model as well as some experimental models based on quality and outcomes.

To become a PCMH, a practice must meet a number of standards, including certification by an organization such as the National Committee for Quality Assurance (NCQA). According to the NCQA, by March 2013, they had recognized 5,700 practices and were receiving about 150 new applications per month.[44]

ACCOUNTABLE CARE ORGANIZATIONS

Accountable Care Organizations (ACOs) are large organizations that integrate primary care, specialty services, and inpatient hospital care. They are very similar to the medical home but expand beyond a single primary care practice to include hospital care and specialty care, etc. They have thus been called "medical neighborhoods."[45]

There were more than 600 ACOs by the end of 2013,[46] with roughly two-thirds covering Medicare or Medicaid patients and one-third privately insured patients. See Chapter 5 for more information about ACOs and the Affordable Care Act. Both ACOs and PCMHs show promise, but it's unclear what their long-term impact will be.

Shortages

PHYSICIAN SHORTAGE

While this section refers to the number of total physicians practicing in the U.S., a shortage can also represent the distribution of physicians in terms of both geography and specialty.

The Association of American Medical Colleges forecasts a shortfall of 91,000 physicians by 2020.[47] We are likely to see significantly increased demand for medical services in the coming years, due in large part to the ACA's major expansion of health insurance coverage as well as a rapidly aging population. In addition, the unequal distribution of physicians throughout the country means some areas are already experiencing a shortage; the federal government already designates more than 20% of the U.S. population as living in a "health professional shortage area."[48] A national consensus is growing that the supply of physicians needs to be expanded, but to do so will require changes to an already controversial system.

In 2013, there were more than 105,000 medical students in the U.S.[49,50] and almost 124,000 resident physicians.[51] (There are more residents than students because many residencies are longer than the four years of medical school and also because many residency slots are filled by international medical graduates.) Many more people would like to become physicians, but the

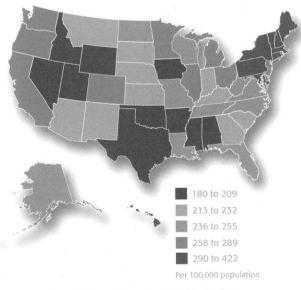

Total Active Physicians per Capita

- 180 to 209
- 213 to 232
- 236 to 255
- 258 to 289
- 290 to 422

Per 100,000 population

Association of American Medical Colleges, "2013 State Physician Workforce Data Book," Nov. 2013.

bottleneck (and barrier) to actually becoming one is the limited number of medical school and *particularly* residency slots, which limits physician supply and contributes to the shortage. See Chapter 6 for more about residency structure and funding.

Arguments can be made both for and against limiting the number of medical students and residents (which is, ultimately, a limit on physicians).

Here's a point–counterpoint summary of the arguments.

Point: Limiting Physician Number is Good	Counterpoint: Limiting Physician Number is Bad
▸ Entering medical students can be assured that, though they're taking on massive debt (a median of $170K per student)[52] they will definitely get jobs when it's all over. ▸ These limits reflect maintenance of high standards by accreditation organizations and medical licensing boards. ▸ The U.S. already has more physicians per capita than it has ever had,[53] and areas of the U.S. with more physicians per capita don't have better health outcomes but do have higher costs and poorer coordination of care.[54] ▸ It would be expensive—and drive up costs further—to fund many new residency programs.	▸ Competition is limited, keeping salaries artificially high. ▸ Standards are too high, blocking students who would make good physicians. ▸ These limits lead to a patient-to-physician ratio that's too high, especially in primary care and in rural areas. ▸ Physicians must put in long hours to compensate for the small workforce, leading to sleep-deprived and overworked physicians. ▸ The U.S. population is aging, and older people require more medical care.

We should note, too, that increasing the number of physicians isn't the only option to address the physician shortage. Alternatives include telemedicine (i.e., physicians "see" patients in remote places through video) and training more Advanced Practice Nurses and Physician Assistants (i.e., "Mid-level providers," see Chapter 6).

NURSING SHORTAGE

There are more than three million registered nurses (RNs) in the U.S., representing the largest sector of health care workers. Hospitals began reporting a shortage of RNs in 1998, with a nadir in 2001—when the media made it sound as if there were only three nurses, and two of them were about to quit. This shortage has lessened in recent years, with an increase in RNs largely attributed to nurses over age 50 and foreign-born nurses, who represent 36% and 16%, respectively, of all nurses.[55]

While the nursing shortage may not be an immediate crisis, it's worth noting that many experts still project an ongoing and increasing shortage in the near future as older nurses retire and the U.S. population continues to grow older.[56] The federal government estimates more than one million[g] nursing job openings over the next 10 years.[57]

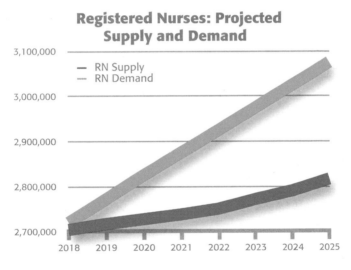

Registered Nurses: Projected Supply and Demand

— RN Supply
— RN Demand

American Hospital Association, "TrendWatch Chartbook," Sept. 2013.
Used with permission. Note: Supply and demand in full-time equivalents.

According to a consortium of leading nursing organizations, the new nursing shortage is evidenced by fewer nurses entering the workforce; acute nursing shortages in certain geographic areas; and a shortage of nurses adequately prepared to meet certain areas of patient need in a changing health care environment.[58] The current, aging nursing population and the declining number of nursing professionals in the academic pipeline indicate that the nursing shortage may only grow more serious as time goes on. Adding to that trend, young, male, and minority (particularly Hispanic) groups are underrepresented in the nursing workforce. In 2010, an estimated 9% of the RN workforce was male and 5% was Hispanic.[59]

g   Yeah, a million.

Finally, no one really knows how the Affordable Care Act and other health care reforms will affect the availability of jobs, salaries, and certification requirements of nurses. Given the incredible importance of RNs in high-quality administration of care, this is a major issue requiring attention.

Hospital-Specific Concerns

Hospitals are huge businesses in addition to being providers of care, and as such they have particular concerns. First, let's hear it from the horse's mouth: What are hospital CEOs concerned about? Here's a graphic showing what 472 hospital CEOs rank as the top issues confronting hospitals in 2013.[60]

Next, we will review a few issues highlighted above in greater detail: "Readmissions under Reform" and "Uncompensated or Undercompensated Care."

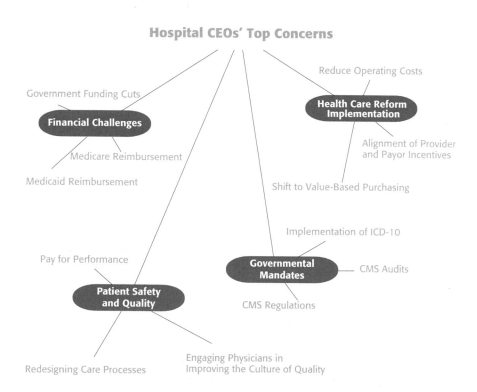

Hospital CEOs' Top Concerns

Reduce Operating Costs

Government Funding Cuts

Health Care Reform Implementation

Financial Challenges

Alignment of Provider and Payor Incentives

Medicare Reimbursement

Medicaid Reimbursement

Shift to Value-Based Purchasing

Implementation of ICD-10

Pay for Performance

Governmental Mandates

CMS Audits

Patient Safety and Quality

CMS Regulations

Redesigning Care Processes

Engaging Physicians in Improving the Culture of Quality

Adapted from: American College of Healthcare Executives, "Top Issues Confronting Hospitals: 2013," Jan. 2014.

READMISSIONS UNDER REFORM

Once a hospital patient no longer needs around-the-clock medical care and is well enough to leave the acute-care setting, she or he can be discharged. The patient has been successfully treated and will not need to be hospitalized again for the same problem. That's the plan, anyway. In reality, many patients are admitted to the hospital again within 30 days of having been discharged; i.e., they are "readmitted." The rate of readmissions for Medicare patients is almost 20%,[61] a level that represents both a serious failure in quality of care and a significant expense to the federal government. Readmission rates also vary significantly from hospital to hospital and by geographic region.

Let's briefly take a look at the numbers, using data from 2010.[61] In that year, 31 million Medicare beneficiaries had 10 million hospital admissions. Of those patients, 1.2 million were readmitted to the hospital within 30 days. While most of these patients were only readmitted once, a smaller subset of 150,000 beneficiaries experienced three or more readmissions. These frequent fliers racked up $116,000 in medical costs annually, more than 10 times what Medicare spends on the average beneficiary.

As you might imagine, Medicare would like to reduce readmissions. The Affordable Care Act included a new financial penalty on hospitals that have "excess readmissions" for patients after acute MI (heart attack), heart failure, or pneumonia (with more conditions to be added in the future). The goal is to financially incentivize hospitals to reduce readmissions and improve their patients' transitions of care. The maximum financial penalty per hospital started at 1% of Medicare reimbursements and is slated to rise to 3% by 2015.

Although those penalties may seem minor at first glance, their effect has been profound and widespread. In 2012, the government penalized more than 2,000 hospitals (two-thirds of all the hospitals they evaluated) for a total of $280 million.[62] Two hundred seventy-six hospitals received the maximum penalty for readmissions, including top-ranked hospitals such as Beth Israel Deaconess Medical Center in Boston, which lost nearly $2 million.[63] Not surprisingly, hospitals are now investing lots of time and money into home visits, patient education, care transitions programs, data analytics, and other strategies to reduce readmissions.[64] Early evidence shows that the national readmission rate for Medicare has declined since the inception of the program,[65] likely showing that the penalties are having some effect.

However, there are many criticisms of the readmissions penalty program. We'll highlight a few here:

▸ Readmission rates are not a good indicator of quality and reducing readmissions may not actually improve health outcomes.[66]

▸ Many readmissions occur for reasons outside the hospitals' control, like patients who don't take (or can't afford) their medications.

▸ Medicare does not adjust penalties for patients' race or socioeconomic status, despite evidence that poor and minority patients have higher readmission rates. Not surprisingly, hospitals that serve the poorest patients are more likely to be penalized.[67]

▸ The penalty is calculated based on "all-cause" readmissions, even if they are unrelated to the original condition (with a few minor exceptions). For example, if a patient treated for pneumonia happens to break his or her leg three weeks later and is brought to the hospital for surgery, that counts as a readmission.[68]

UNCOMPENSATED OR UNDERCOMPENSATED CARE

Uncompensated care and undercompensated care are major problems for many hospitals. Uncompensated care includes both charity care (which the hospital gives away for free and doesn't expect to recover) and bad debt (which the hospital tries to recover from patients, who are often un- or under-insured). In 2012, U.S. hospitals reported $45.9 billion in uncompensated care, which made up 6.1% of their total expenses. This amount has increased ten-fold in the past 20 years, though the percentage has remained steady.[69]

As the American Hospital Association (AHA) states, "Payment rates for Medicare and Medicaid, with the exception of managed care plans, are set by law rather than through a negotiation process as with private insurers. These payment rates are currently set below the costs of providing care, resulting in underpayment."[70] In 2012, the AHA found, Medicare compensated only 86% of costs, and Medicaid compensated only 89% of costs; combined, this made up $56 billion in lost revenue.[70] Previously, it was thought that such funding cuts by public insurance were simply "shifted" to private insurance. The evidence, though, argues against cost-shifting. One recent study found that when Medicare lowers payments by 10%, private insurance payments also fall by 3–8%.[71]

Hospitals likely make up for this lost income by increasing volume and slimming operations. How to evaluate such changes (which may include mergers and cutting staff) depends on the specifics, but it's important to note that decreasing payments may lead to unforeseen consequences down the line.

THE HOSPITAL–PHYSICIAN RELATIONSHIP

Most of the physicians who provide inpatient care aren't actually hospital employees. Hospital–physician relationships developed in a time when physicians were their own bosses. When a patient was too sick to be treated as an outpatient, the physician would admit the patient to a local hospital, where he or she would direct the patient's care. Upon discharge, the patient received two separate bills—one from the physician for the care received and another from the hospital for use of a bed, supplies, and hospital staff.

Traditionally, physicians operated as independent contractors, and hospitals contracted with them in one of several ways, including:

- ▸ Independent physicians who worked primarily in outpatient settings could maintain privileges to admit their patients to one or more hospitals.
- ▸ Multiple physicians aligned to offer their services together as a "medical group;" one or more hospitals/health care networks then contracted with the group to provide patient care in their facilities.
- ▸ At some academic medical centers, physicians were employed by a medical school or academic physician organization and maintained an exclusive contract with an affiliated hospital.

For any of these relationships, all of which are still common today, physicians order and use hospital resources (i.e., spend hospital money) without being directly employed by the hospital (the usual way that employers exert control over their employees). The upshot is that hospitals may have to use different methods than a traditional employer to influence physician behavior—behavior that has far-reaching effects on many health care issues, such as cost control and quality improvement.

However, this traditional hospital–physician relationship is evolving. A small percentage of physicians have historically been hospital employees— emergency physicians, pathologists, and, more recently, hospitalists, for example—but today, a growing number of physicians in all specialties are eschewing their traditional independence in favor of direct employment by a hospital, health care network, or insurance company. One large example is Kaiser Permanente, a California-based HMO (read about HMOs in Chapter 2) that directly employs physicians. For other hospitals, many of the physicians they employ are hospitalists who only treat hospitalized patients and don't maintain an outpatient clinic.

References

1. Department of Veteran Affairs. VHA Facility Quality and Safety Report—Fiscal Year 2012 Data. www.va.gov/HEALTH/docs/VHA_Quality_and_Safety_Report_2013.pdf. Accessed June 13, 2014.
2. Asch SM, McGlynn EA, et al. Comparison of Quality of Care for Patients in the Veterans Health Administration and Patients in a National Sample. *Annals of Internal Medicine.* 2004;141(12):938.
3. American Hospital Association. Fast Facts on US Hospitals. www.aha.org/research/rc/stat-studies/fast-facts.shtml. Accessed June 9, 2014.
4. Anderson K, Gevas G. The Tax Status of Not-for-Profit Hospitals under Siege & the Financial Implications of Recent Attacks. Vol 2011: National City; 2006.
5. ACLU. Miscarriage of Medicine: The Growth of Catholic Hospitals and the Threat to Reproductive Health Care. 2014. www.aclu.org/religion-belief-reproductive-freedom/miscarriage-medicine-growth-catholic-hospitals-and-threat.
6. Hospital Corporation of America. About Our Company. hcahealthcare.com/about/. Accessed June 9, 2014.
7. Rau J. Doctor-Owned Hospitals Prosper under Health Law. www.kaiserhealthnews.org/stories/2013/april/12/doctor-owned-hospitals-quality-bonuses.aspx. Accessed June 9, 2014.
8. Iglehart JK. The Emergence of Physician-Owned Specialty Hospitals. *New England Journal of Medicine.* 2005;352(1):78.
9. Association of American Medical Colleges. Teaching Hospitals. www.aamc.org/about/membership/378786/teachinghospitals.html. Accessed June 16 2014.
10. Children's Hospital Association. History of Children's Hospitals. www.childrenshospitals.net/AM/Template.cfm?Section=Facts_and_Trends&CONTENTID=12693&TEMPLATE=/CM/ContentDisplay.cfm. Accessed June 9, 2014.
11. Shriners Hospitals for Children. www.shrinershospitalsforchildren.org/. Accessed June 9, 2014.
12. National Center for Health Statistics. Health, United States, 2012 with Special Feature on Emergency Care. www.cdc.gov/nchs/data/hus/hus12.pdf. Accessed June 9, 2014.
13. MEDPAC. March 2014 Report to the Congress: Medicare Payment Policy,. www.medpac.gov/documents/mar14_entirereport.pdf. Accessed June 10, 2014.
14. National Association of Community Health Centers. About Our Health Centers. www.nachc.org/about-our-health-centers.cfm. Accessed June 13, 2014.
15. Beitsch LM, Brooks RG, et al. Public Health at Center Stage: New Roles, Old Props. *Health Affairs.* 2006;25(4):911.
16. Weinick R, Bristol S, et al. Urgent Care Centers in the U.S.: Findings from a National Survey. *BMC Health Services Research.* 2009;9(1):79.
17. Urgent Care Center. Urgent Care Press. www.urgentcarecenter.org/press.html. Accessed June 28, 2014.
18. Merchant Medicine. Taking Medicine to the Marketplace. www.merchantmedicine.com/Home.cfm?view=Retail. Accessed June 9, 2014.

19. Hechcock B. Ambulatory Surgery Centers Catching up to Hospitals, *Dallas Business Journal*. www.bizjournals.com/dallas/news/2013/01/29/ambulatory-surgery-centers-catching-up.html. Accessed June 23, 2014.

20. Cullen KA, Hall MJ, et al. *Ambulatory Surgery in the United States, 2006.* US Dept. of Health and Human Services, Centers for Disease Control and Prevention, National Center for Health Statistics; 2009.

21. Hollingsworth JM, Ye Z, et al. Physician-Ownership of Ambulatory Surgery Centers Linked to Higher Volume of Surgeries. *Health Affairs.* 2010;29(4):683.

22. The National Association for Home Care and Hospice. Basic Statistics About Home Care. www.nahc.org/assets/1/7/10HC_Stats.pdf. Accessed June 23, 2014.

23. Caregiver Action Network. Caregiving Statistics. caregiveraction.org/statistics/. Accessed June 16, 2014.

24. Feinberg L, Reinhard SC, et al. Valuing the Invaluable: 2011 Update—the Growing Contributions and Costs of Family Caregiving. assets.aarp.org/rgcenter/ppi/ltc/i51-caregiving.pdf. Accessed June 9, 2014.

25. National Hospice and Palliative Care Organization. Nhpco Facts and Figures on Hospice Care. www.nhpco.org/sites/default/files/public/Statistics_Research/2012_Facts_Figures.pdf. Accessed June 23, 2014.

26. Connor SR, Pyenson B, et al. Comparing Hospice and Nonhospice Patient Survival among Patients Who Die within a Three-Year Window. *Journal of pain and symptom management.* 2007;33(3):238.

27. Nahin RL, Barnes PM, et al. Costs of Complementary and Alternative Medicine (CAM) and Frequency of Visits to Cam Practitioners: United States, 2007. *National health statistics reports.* 2009;18.

28. Health Resources and Services Administration. The Physician Workforce: Projections and Research into Current Issues Affecting Supply and Demand. bhpr.hrsa.gov/healthworkforce/reports/physwfissues.pdf. Accessed June 7, 2014.

29. Agency for Healthcare Research and Quality. Primary Care Workforce Facts and Stats. www.ahrq.gov/research/findings/factsheets/primary/pcworkforce/index.html. Accessed June 9, 2014.

30. Yarnall KS, Pollak KI, et al. Primary Care: Is There Enough Time for Prevention? *Am J Public Health.* Apr 2003;93(4):635.

31. Ostby T, Yarnall KS, et al. Is There Time for Management of Patients with Chronic Diseases in Primary Care? *Ann Fam Med.* May 2005;3(3):209.

32. Stange KC, Zyzanski SJ, et al. Illuminating the 'Black Box'. A Description of 4454 Patient Visits to 138 Family Physicians. *The Journal of family practice.* May 1998;46(5):377.

33. Weida NA, Phillips Jr RL, et al. Graham Center Policy One-Pager: Loss of Primary Care Residency Positions Amidst Growth in Other Specialties. *Am Fam Physician.* 2010;82(2):121.

34. Health Resources and Service Administration. Designated Health Professional Shortage Areas Statistics. ersrs.hrsa.gov/reportserver/Pages/ReportViewer.aspx?/HGDW_Reports/BCD_HPSA/BCD_HPSA_SCR50_Smry_HTML&rs:Format=HTML4.0. Accessed June 23, 2014.

35. Starfield B, Shi L, et al. Contribution of Primary Care to Health Systems and Health. *Milbank Quarterly.* 2005;83(3):457.

36. Bodenheimer T, Pham HH. Primary Care: Current Problems and Proposed Solutions. *Health Affairs.* 2010;29(5):799.

37. Kletke PR, Emmons DW, et al. Current Trends in Physicians' Practice Arrangements. From Owners to Employees. *JAMA: The Journal of the American Medical Association.* 1996;276(7):555.

38. Kane C. Policy Research Perspectives: The Practice Arrangements of Patient Care Physicians, 2007-2008: An Analysis by Age Cohort and Gender. Vol 2011: American Medical Association; 2009.

39. Moses H, Matheson D, et al. The Anatomy of Health Care in the United States. *JAMA: The Journal of the American Medical Association.* 2013/11/13 2013;310(18):1947.

40. Rundall TG, Davies HT, et al. Doctor-Manager Relationships in the United States and the United Kingdom. *Journal of healthcare management / American College of Healthcare Executives.* 2004;49(4):251.

41. Jensen E, Mendonca L. Why America Spends More on Health Care. nihcm.org/pdf/EV_JensenMendonca_FINAL.pdf. Accessed June 9, 2014.

42. Agency for Healthcare Research and Quality. Defining the PCMH. pcmh.ahrq.gov/page/defining-pcmh. Accessed June 10, 2014.

43. Erickson SM. The Patient Centered Medical Home: Overview of the Model and Movement Part I. www.acponline.org/running_practice/delivery_and_payment_models/pcmh/understanding/erickson1.pdf. Accessed June 10, 2014.

44. National Committee for Quality Assurance. Patient-Centered Medical Homes. www.ncqa.org/Portals/0/Public%20Policy/2013%20PDFS/pcmh%202011%20fact%20sheet.pdf. Accessed June 10, 2014.

45. Fisher ES. Building a Medical Neighborhood for the Medical Home. *New England Journal of Medicine.* Sep 2008;359(12):1202.

46. Petersen M, Gardner P, et al. Growth and Dispersion of Accountable Care Organizations: June 2014 Update. leavittpartners.com/wp-content/uploads/2014/06/Growth-and-Dispersion-of-Accountable-Care-Organizations-June2014.pdf. Accessed June 28, 2014.

47. Association of American Medical Colleges. Physician Shortages to Worsen without Increases in Residency Training. www.aamc.org/download/286592/data/. Accessed June 9, 2014.

48. Kirch DG, Vernon DJ. Confronting the Complexity of the Physician Workforce Equation. *JAMA: The Journal of the American Medical Association.* 2008;299(22):2680.

49. Osteopathic Medical Profession. Annual Statistics. www.osteopathic.org/inside-aoa/about/aoa-annual-statistics/Documents/2013-OMP-report.pdf. Accessed June 10, 2014.

50. Association of American Medical Colleges. 2013 Facts Table. www.aamc.org/download/321526/data/2013factstable26-2.pdf. Accessed June 10, 2014.

51. American Osteopathic Association. Accreditation Release. www.acgme.org/acgmeweb/portals/0/PDFS/Nasca-Community/SingleAccreditationRelease2-26.pdf. Accessed June 23, 2014.

52. Association of American Medical Colleges. Medical Student Education: Debt, Costs, and Loan Repayment Fact Card. www.aamc.org/download/152968/data/debtfactcard.pdf. Accessed June 9, 2014.

53. Kliff S. We Have More Doctors Per Capita Than Ever Before. *The Washington Post.* 2011-12-16.

54. Goodman DC, Fisher ES. Physician Workforce Crisis? Wrong Diagnosis, Wrong Prescription. *New England Journal of Medicine.* 2008;358(16):1658.

55. Buerhaus PI, Auerbach DI, et al. The Recent Surge in Nurse Employment: Causes and Implications. *Health Affairs.* 2009-07-01 2009;28(4):657.

56. McMenamin P. RN Retirements—Tsunami Warning! : Nursingworld.org; 2014.

57. Bureau of Labor Statistics. Employment Projections: 2012-2022 Summary. www.bls.gov/news.release/ecopro.nr0.htm. Accessed June 10, 2014.

58. American Association of Colleges of Nursing. Strategies to Reverse the New Nursing Shortage. www.aacn.nche.edu/publications/position/tri-council-shortage. Accessed April 24, 2014.

59. National Center for Health Workforce Analysis. The U.S. Nursing Workforce: Trends in Supply and Education. bhpr.hrsa.gov/healthworkforce/reports/nursingworkforce/nursingworkforcefullreport.pdf. Accessed June 28, 2014.

60. American College of Healthcare. Healthcare Executives Announce Top Issues Confronting Hospitals: 2012. www.ache.org/Pubs/Releases/2013/Top-Issues-Confronting-Hospitals-2012.cfm. Accessed June 10, 2014.

61. Centers for Medicare & Medicaid Services. National Medicare Readmission Findings: Recent Data and Trends. www.academyhealth.org/files/2012/sunday/brennan.pdf. Accessed June 23, 2014.

62. Rau J. Medicare Revises Readmissions Penalties—Again. www.kaiserhealthnews.org/stories/2013/march/14/revised-readmissions-statistics-hospitals-medicare.aspx. Accessed June 10, 2014.

63. Conaboy C. Hospitals Look to Lower Readmission Rates in Face of Penalties. www.boston.com/lifestyle/health/2012/11/12/hospitals-look-lower-readmission-rates-face-penalties/OcT0EZRe4PK3Q5JzHEIGNP/story.html. Accessed June 9, 2014.

64. Rau J. Hospitals Offer Wide Array of Services to Keep Patients from Needing to Return. www.kaiserhealthnews.org/Stories/2012/November/28/hospital-services-to-reduce-readmissions.aspx. Accessed June 23, 2014.

65. Centers for Medicare & Medicaid Services. New Data Shows Affordable Care Act Reforms Are Leading to Lower Hospital Readmission Rates for Medicare Beneficiaries. blog.cms.gov/2013/12/06/new-data-shows-affordable-care-act-reforms-are-leading-to-lower-hospital-readmission-rates-for-medicare-beneficiaries/. Accessed June 9, 2014.

66. American College of Cardiology. 30-Day Readmission: A Lousy Quality Metric in HF? www.cardiosource.org/News-Media/Publications/CardioSource-World-News/2013/August/30-Day-Readmission-A-Lousy-Quality-Metric-in-HF.aspx. Accessed June 10, 2014.

67. James J. Health Policy Brief: Medicare Hospital Readmissions Reduction Program. *Health Affairs.* 2013.

68. American College of Emergency Physicians. Medicare's Hospital Readmission Reduction Program FAQ. www.acep.org/Legislation-and-Advocacy/Practice-Management-Issues/Physician-Payment-Reform/Medicare-s-Hospital-Readmission-Reduction-Program-FAQ/. Accessed June 10, 2014.

69. American Hospital Association. Uncompensated Hospital Care Cost Fact Sheet. www.aha.org/content/14/14uncompensatedcare.pdf. Accessed June 28, 2014.

70. American Hospital Association. Underpayment by Medicare and Medicaid Fact Sheet. www.aha.org/content/14/2012-medicare-med-underpay.pdf. Accessed June 28, 2014.

71. White C. Contrary to Cost-Shift Theory, Lower Medicare Hospital Payment Rates for Inpatient Care Lead to Lower Private Payment Rates. *Health Affairs.* 2013-05-01 May 2013;32(5):935.

Chapter 2
Insurance and Economics

If you want to understand the health care system, it's essential to understand insurance and economics—but being essential doesn't mean it's easy. We know these topics can be confusing and convoluted, as does anyone who's tried to purchase health insurance or understand why health care costs so dang much. So we've done our best to reduce the abstractions and confusion, because the secret is that the economics of health care is fascinating. Once you begin to understand it, you'll see how patients' and providers' behavior that seems to have nothing to do with money ends up affecting the bottom line and how the structure of the U.S. health care system influences that behavior.

Everything about health care discussed in Chapter 1 costs money, and money changes options, affects behavior, and produces problems. Insurance—the way we pay for care—and economics—the study of the production, distribution, and consumption of that care—help to piece together what the problems are, what causes them, and how to fix them.

Health Economics 101

Before throwing you into the health economics deep end, we want to give a little economics background for those not already familiar with it. So if you *are* familiar with it, feel free to skip this section. If not, here's your swimming lesson!

What Is Insurance and Why Have It?

Your auto insurance doesn't pay for tune-ups, but it *will* pay for your car if it's totaled in a wreck. Life involves a certain amount of luck, and accidental events often come with big price tags. Insurance, then, exists to defray the potentially devastating expenses you may or may not find yourself up against in life, vehicular or otherwise.

The logic behind insurance is two-fold. First, money should be set aside in small increments over time to spread out the potential cost of an unexpected large expense. Second, your money should be pooled with others' money to further spread out large costs. The benefit to insured individuals is that, as long as you make monthly payments, your accidents are covered—even if you get into a wreck after holding the policy for a week. The benefit to the insurance company is that it gets to keep your monthly payments if that wreck never happens. The benefit to society is that a few car crashes seem more trivial when the costs are spread out among thousands of people.

As a metaphor, though, comparing health insurance to auto insurance is an obvious over-simplification. As we said, health care is complicated! This metaphor ignores important differences between auto and health insurance. Most fundamentally, a car is not equivalent to a body. Having a crappy car is, in some sense, both a choice and not that big of a deal. On the other hand, having an injured or sick body may be due, at least in part, to genetics or how you were raised or the environment where you live. Further, even if your behavior may have played a role in substandard health, society's values make us wary of simply making people live with the severe consequences of illness and death. Our health is a much bigger deal than any car could ever be.

In all types of health insurance, the following parties exist: patients (or consumers, depending on your perspective), providers (physicians, nurses, etc.), and payors. These three parties have varying incentives with regard to cost, access, and quality, and these incentives may not always align.

Economic Terms

INFORMATION ASYMMETRY

As a concept, this is as simple as it sounds: One side of a transaction has more information than the other side, which is usually the case for patients and providers, or patients and payors. Information asymmetry influences a wide swath of interactions in the health care system. It often involves situations in which one side wants the other side to act on its behalf. For example, the insurance company wants the policyholder to incur fewer costs (whether through good health or through forgoing medical services) so the company won't have to pay. Information asymmetry can cause moral hazard, adverse selection, and conflict of interest, all of which are explained below.

MORAL HAZARD

Let's say you fall in love with a house on the beach, but it happens to sit on a stretch of the coast known for getting beaten in hurricane after hurricane. "That's too bad," you think, "but I guess insurance would pay for it," and you buy it anyway. That's moral hazard: the trend toward more risky behavior when you know you won't end up having to cover the full cost.

Examples of moral hazard in medicine include smoking and neglecting to get regular check-ups because you know that large cost consequences down the line will be covered by insurance. Many think that moral hazard plays a big role in rising health care costs, and things like co-pays, co-insurance, and deductibles exist to reduce its effects by making patients pay for some portion of the care they receive.

ADVERSE SELECTION

Contrast a healthy 22-year-old who runs 20 miles a week with a 45-year-old diabetic who had a heart attack five years ago. Which one is more likely to desire health insurance?

Insurance exists to spread costs among even those who don't end up incurring them. The law mandates that those who have cars must get auto insurance, so it's easy to spread costs among the population, but the same hasn't historically been true with health insurance. Young, healthy people have low enough risk that they can eliminate costs entirely by not purchasing insurance. The risk-spreading purpose of insurance is thus compromised, as the total number of people paying premiums goes down while the number of people making claims stays the same. Thus, premiums grow untenably high for remaining policyholders. That's adverse selection. (This concept is a key reason for the individual mandate. See Chapter 5 for more information.)

BEHAVIORAL ECONOMICS

Humans are not perfectly rational beings. What's more, unlike in models of behavior used in classical economics, we aren't motivated solely by money. We make imperfect risk-benefit analyses, respond to the heat of the moment, and ignore evidence to the contrary of our beliefs and desires—so a person might end up gambling instead of saving for retirement, punching his best friend during a brief argument, and buying a gas guzzler despite high gas prices. Behavioral economics takes this irrationality into account as a combination of both economics and psychology—a study of how humans actually behave in the world. Researchers are now using behavioral economics to study thorny health issues like obesity and medication adherence.

Health Insurance Basics

An individual enrolled in a health insurance plan or policy is known as a **beneficiary** or member. The person who purchases the insurance is the subscriber, and any other people on the policy (spouse or children) are dependents. The insurance company charges the subscriber a monthly fee, called the **premium**. When a beneficiary receives health care services, the insurance company will pay the health care provider, clinic, or hospital on behalf of the beneficiary. However, the beneficiary is still required to pay for some of the cost that he or she incurs—this is known as **cost sharing.** Cost sharing comes in different flavors:

▸ The **deductible** is a fixed-dollar annual amount of health care costs that the beneficiary must pay entirely out of pocket. For example, if the deductible is $500, the first $500 in medical costs incurred each year is paid by the beneficiary; for costs beyond $500, the insurance company may pay completely or require a co-payment or co-insurance.

▸ A **co-payment (or "co-pay")** is a fixed-dollar amount that the beneficiary must pay for certain services. For example, the policy might say that the beneficiary pays $15 out of pocket for each primary care visit and $25 for each specialist visit, while the insurance company pays the rest of the bill.

▸ **Co-insurance** is similar to co-payment, but it's a percentage of the bill rather than a fixed amount. For example, the beneficiary might pay 20% of the cost of a primary care visit and 25% of the cost of a specialist visit, and the insurance company pays the rest.

▸ The **out-of-pocket max** is the total amount that the beneficiary must pay in a given year. This includes what the beneficiary pays toward the deductible, any co-pays, or co-insurance. After that total amount has been reached, the insurer pays 100% of the costs for all covered services.

Legal regulation of health insurance is a bit messier. Some insurance plans, like self-insured employers and Medicare, are federally regulated. Others, such as plans bought individually, are governed primarily by state law. Insurance regulations vary significantly state by state, so while we'll discuss the fundamentals of health insurance here, keep in mind that the specifics depend on the state where the beneficiary lives.

Insurance

Coverage and Organization Formats

Indemnity plans were both the simplest and the most popular type of insurance plans for most of the 20th century. The best known of these plans were those offered by Blue Cross/Blue Shield. In an indemnity (or "conventional") plan, the beneficiary has a fixed amount of cost-sharing regardless of which physician or hospital he or she visits. Beneficiaries are responsible for paying premiums to the insurer and co-insurance (after the deductible has been reached) to the provider or facility, while the insurance company reimburses the provider or facility for the majority of the bill.

As health care spending skyrocketed throughout the 1980s, many insurance companies moved to a new model—the **Managed Care Organization (MCO)**—in an attempt to constrain costs. As the name implies, these insurers take a more active role in managing the *care* their beneficiaries receive (and thus the costs they incur), rather than focusing solely on premiums and reimbursements. Indemnity plans have little leverage to influence provider prices or what care their beneficiaries receive. Managed care plans stress the integration of insurance and medical care, especially by exerting more control over providers and patients regarding reimbursements and care utilization.

The original MCO is the **Health Management Organization (HMO),** the most tightly integrated insurance plan. Beneficiaries of HMO plans can only receive covered care from physicians in the HMO "network."[a] In some plans, these physicians are directly employed by the HMO; in others, the physicians are still in private practice (page 8) or part of another sort of clinic or hospital-based group but sign contracts with the HMO, becoming "participating providers." HMOs also emphasize primary care, usually requiring the member to get a referral from his or her PCP (primary care provider) for specialty services, a practice known as "gatekeeping." Some hospitalizations and costly outpatient procedures will only be covered if the insurance company "pre-authorizes" them in advance.

The above paragraph introduces three much reviled practices: restricting provider choice, gatekeeping, and pre-authorization. Patients generally hate this stuff, but insurance companies do it because it keeps costs down. HMOs were successful in bringing down health care spending in the 1990s but faced a major backlash from patients, providers, and lawmakers who felt that the insurance companies had gone too far in restricting choice. Thousands of state laws were passed to regulate HMOs, which reduced some of their power to restrain utilization and spending. Nationwide, the number of individuals enrolled in HMOs has decreased significantly in the past 15 years.

Preferred Provider Organizations (PPOs) negotiate contracts with physicians, who form the plan's network. These physicians agree to charge discounted rates to the plan's beneficiaries in exchange for the increased

---

a   Patients can still visit providers, clinics, or hospitals that aren't in the HMO network, but must pay the bill out-of-pocket.

flow of patients from participating in the network. Beneficiaries can receive care from providers who aren't in the network, but when the services are obtained out-of-network, the beneficiary has a higher deductible and has higher co-insurance and co-payments to make. The insurer's goal is to create incentives to keep the beneficiary using in-network providers. PPOs place less emphasis on coordination of care and don't employ gatekeeping or capitation. Without gatekeeping, and with the ability of members to receive covered care out-of-network, PPOs offer beneficiaries more choices, but the insurers don't have as much power as HMOs to constrain spending.

The final MCO plan is the **Point of Service (POS),** which combines features of HMOs and PPOs. POS plans were very popular in the 1990s but have largely been supplanted by PPOs, because requirements for authorization before seeing a specialist have proven to be highly unpopular.

Consumer-Driven Health Plans are a relatively new type of coverage that give beneficiaries more choice and control over their health care spending. Think of these as tax-free bank accounts that can only be used for medical expenses (non-medical withdrawals incur penalties). They come in several formats—health savings accounts (HSA), flexible spending accounts

Distribution of Health Plan Enrollment for Covered Workers, by Plan Type

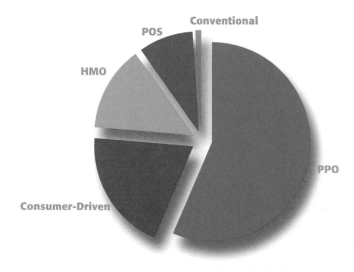

The Henry J. Kaiser Family Foundation, "Employer Health Benefits 2013 Annual Survey," August 2013. Used with permission.

(FSA), and health reimbursement accounts (HRA). HSAs were first developed in 2003 as a way for individuals to opt out of traditional insurance. Patients who use these are partially saving for their own health needs rather than just paying insurers monthly; however, those who enroll in an HSA must also enroll in an insurance plan with high deductibles (between $1,250–$6,250 for individuals and $2,500–$12,500 for families).[1] HSAs are of primary benefit to patients who are young, healthy, and expect a steady source of income, and the plans allow members of this population to lower their spending to match their low risk.

Premiums—How Are They Set?

In any insurance company, over the course of time, expenses will equal the amount of care the company has to pay for plus administrative costs. To stay solvent, the amount the company takes in from monthly premiums needs to equal these expenses.

Obviously, though, not all people who purchase insurance will cost the company the same amount. In America, the sickest 5% of the population accounts for 50% of total health care spending, while the healthiest half of the population only accounts for 3% of health care spending.[2] Historically, insurance companies could take these discrepancies into account when setting premiums. Individual customers were subject to "medical underwriting," or the practice of estimating how much medical care an individual is likely to need and charging a rate based on that (so the sicker you are, the higher premium you pay). Contrast this practice with the practice used for insurance you get through your employer: Every employee pays the same amount, regardless of their medical history; this is called a "community rating." In community rating, the premium cost is calculated by dividing the total expenses by the number of beneficiaries.

The Affordable Care Act changes medical underwriting to make it more like community rating. As of 2014, insurance companies no longer can take past medical history into account for medical underwriting; they can only adjust rates based on:
- Age
- Geographic location
- Family composition (i.e., number of children)
- Tobacco use

See Chapter 5 for much more information on new insurance rating rules.

Your premiums are paying for two things:
1. Benefit pay-out (yours *and* others)
2. Running the insurance company

There is a trade-off between premiums and benefits; generally, the more you pay monthly, the better benefits you get. That's one thing you are paying for: lower co-pays, lower deductible, better coverage. But your premium dollars aren't earmarked just for you. They go into a pool to pay out *all* benefit coverage; thus, your premiums go up as the pool of other insured folks gets more expensive.

And, as with any business, your premiums must cover the cost of running the company, i.e., overhead. In health insurance, there is a term for this: the medical loss ratio (MLR). The MLR is the percentage of insurance premiums that the insurance company spends on clinical services and activities to improve quality.[3] Put in plain English, this is the percentage of your insurance premium that actually pays for health care. The rest of the revenue pays for administrative costs, marketing, salaries, overhead, and company profits. For understandable reasons, insurance companies do consider paying for health care to be a loss.

As of 2009, the MLR for the five largest for-profit insurance companies was in the 70% range for individuals and in the 80% range for small and large groups.[4] The Affordable Care Act now requires insurers to keep MLR at 85% for large group insurers and 80% for small group insurers.

Ways to Get Insurance

THROUGH EMPLOYMENT

The current relationship between health insurance and employment arose during World War II after the federal government enacted a freeze on wage increases in private industry. In response, employers improved their non-wage benefits, including health insurance, for employees and their families. This arrangement of employer-sponsored insurance (ESI) spread even more rapidly when the IRS ruled that employer payments for insurance weren't taxable.[5] ESI has since become the predominant method of

Health Insurance in the U.S.

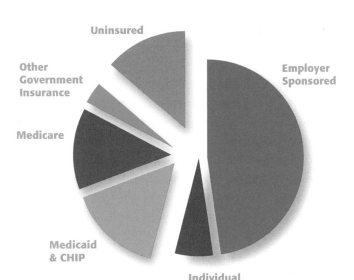

Centers for Medicare & Medicaid Services, "National Health Expenditure Data," Jan. 2014.

obtaining insurance in the U.S.; in 2012, 55% of all insured non-elderly Americans had ESI[6] (down from 70% in 2009), either through their own employer or through a family member.

ESI comes in one of two types, depending on who is assuming the risk for the health care expenses of the covered employees and their families.

Fully Insured: The employer buys insurance from a private insurance company for its employees. In this arrangement, the insurance company is the payor and takes the risk for future medical costs for the beneficiaries. The employer usually works with a broker to price different insurance options—different kinds of plans and from different insurers—and the employee can select from one of these employer-approved plans.

Most plans will also cover spouse and dependents for an increased price, though they are not required to. Premiums are otherwise the same for each employee.[b] The employer contributes 50–90% of the monthly premium, and

---

b   ESI premiums may (depending on state law) be adjusted by the insurer to account for the claims history of the employer, so an employer with a track record of employees who need lots of medical care may have to pay a higher premium. Thus, insurance for employees of mining companies is usually more expensive than those of a health food store.

the employee pays the rest. Employees see reduced wages, as employers must pay less in wages to maintain this benefit; however, neither employees nor employers have to pay income tax on benefits. Thus, though employees have reduced wages, they receive a larger total compensation package.

Self-Insured: If large enough, the employer will often choose to act as the payor and assume the risk of future medical expenses for its own employees. A private insurance company is contracted only to handle the plan's day-to-day administration. The employer also usually purchases what's called "stop loss insurance" from a private insurer, which protects the employer from unexpectedly high costs from employees' medical care. Employees are still required to contribute monthly fees for the cost of their insurance coverage, but the payments go primarily to the employer rather than to the insurance company. Employee enrollment in self-insured plans has continued to rise even as enrollment in ESI in general has fallen.[7,8]

Pros and Cons of ESI

From the employee's standpoint, ESI provides both advantages and disadvantages. The advantages are reduced premiums (due to both the contribution of the employer as well as the economy of scale), and reduced income taxes. The disadvantages are that it reduces your salary and may constrict choice (since you can only choose an insurance plan that's been selected by your employer).[c]

From the insurance company's standpoint, ESI reduces both the need for marketing and adverse selection. A group of employees is likely to be both large (meaning a dependable stream of revenue as long as they maintain a relationship with the employer) and relatively healthy[d] (meaning they won't require as much pay-out on their premiums). While employers do have the clout to reduce premiums from what individual consumers pay, this is still a profitable trade-off for the insurers.

From the employer's standpoint, the advantages of ESI increase with the size of the business. For a large business, the economy of scale means they have to pay less, as a percentage of payroll, to provide the benefit. The

---

c   Historically, ESI has represented another HUGE advantage to employees: You were guaranteed coverage even with a pre-existing condition (on the flip side, that made employees dependent on their jobs and reluctant to switch if it meant losing insurance). However, after 2014, the Affordable Care Act makes it illegal to use pre-existing conditions to deny coverage, so all Americans will enjoy this benefit, regardless of ESI.
d   Compared to a similar-sized group of unemployed individuals.

opposite is true for small employers. You can see this reflected in the number of large companies (>200 workers) vs. small companies (<200 workers) who, pre-2014, provided health insurance: 99% vs. 57%.[9] No matter the employer's size, benefits get increasingly difficult to provide as health costs rise faster than wages. Between 1999 and 2010, health premiums rose by 138%, and wages rose 42%.[10] As a result, before the Affordable Care Act, ESI had been on the decline: From 2001 to 2005, the number of employers providing health insurance decreased from 84% to 80%,[11] and, from 2000 to 2011, the number of working-aged adults receiving ESI decreased from 69% to 58%.[12] Of course, that trend is disrupted by the Affordable Care Act, which includes an "employer mandate" for businesses employing 50+ people to provide insurance. See Chapter 5 for more information.

From society's standpoint, ESI is beneficial in that it can insure a large number of citizens without the government directly insuring them. It's problematic, though, because of the ESI tax subsidy (workers pay taxes only on their wages, not their benefits). Since ESI is paid with pre-tax dollars, that means that (a) society misses out on those taxes (about $250 *billion* each year![13]),

Family Coverage Through ESI: Average Premium Contributions for Employee and Employer

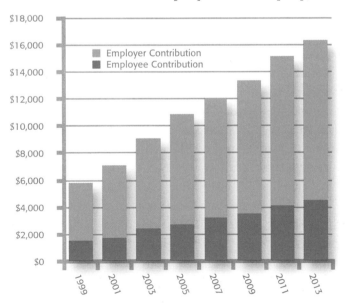

The Henry J. Kaiser Family Foundation, "Employer Health Benefits 2013 Annual Survey," August 2013. Used with permission.

and (b) those with ESI get more bang for their buck, which is unfair to those who purchase insurance outside of employment. Thus, the ESI tax subsidy is an important focus of policy reformers. See Chapter 5 for more information.

PUBLIC INSURANCE PROGRAMS

Thirty-one percent of Americans receive health insurance through one of the following government programs: Medicare, Medicaid, Children's Health Insurance Program (CHIP), Tricare (for active duty military), or the Veterans Health Administration (for veterans).[14] Let's go through these programs.

Medicare

Medicare is a federal program established in 1965 to insure the elderly and some disabled individuals. It is the largest insurer in the nation—meaning the policies Medicare sets have an enormous impact on how health care is run in general.

▸ **Eligibility**

The primary purpose of Medicare is to cover the elderly, though it has been slightly expanded over the years. To be eligible for coverage, a person must:

   ▸ Be at least 65 years old, have been a U.S. citizen or permanent resident for more than five years, and have (or have a spouse who has) paid Medicare taxes for at least 10 years;

   ▸ Be under age 65, be permanently disabled, and have received Social Security disability benefits for at least the previous two years;

   ▸ Be under age 65 and receive Social Security disability benefits for amyotrophic lateral sclerosis (ALS or Lou Gehrig's disease);

   ▸ Be under age 65 and need continuous dialysis or a kidney transplant; or

   ▸ Be under age 65 and have developed health conditions following environmental hazard exposure in an emergency declaration area after June 17, 2009.

▸ **Coverage**

Medicare has four parts:

   ▸ **Part A:** Inpatient insurance, covering stays in hospitals and nursing homes, home health visits, and hospice. These benefits, however, have a limit on the number of days they will pay for in a facility, and they are subject to co-pays and deductibles.

‣ **Part B:** Outpatient insurance, including coverage for physician services, preventive services, and home health visits. These benefits are also subject to co-pays and deductibles.

‣ **Part C:** Also called Medicare Advantage, it allows beneficiaries to enroll in a private insurance plan (like an outside HMO), which will cover all regular Medicare benefits and may cover more or require reduced co-pays and deductibles. Medicare pays these private insurers a fixed amount per month, per beneficiary. About 30% of Medicare beneficiaries are enrolled in a Medicare Advantage plan.[15]

‣ **Part D:** Added in 2005, this is a prescription drug benefit. Part D is voluntary and operates through contracted private insurers. The program is subsidized, particularly for low-income beneficiaries. Previously there existed a "donut hole," causing certain beneficiaries to lose coverage of most of their prescriptions, but the Affordable Care Act "closes" the gap through subsidies and rebates. See Chapter 5 for more information.

‣ **Supplemental Insurance**

Medicare requires somewhat high co-pays and deductibles, doesn't have a limit on out-of-pocket costs, and doesn't pay for long-term care (e.g., a permanent nursing home), eye services, or dental services. Thus, many beneficiaries want additional insurance to reduce their out-of-pocket expenses. Options include:

‣ Employer-sponsored retirement benefits

‣ Medigap: Voluntary insurance offered by private insurers to cover services not included in Medicare Parts A and B (You can't have this with Medicare Advantage.)[16]

‣ Medicaid

‣ **Funding**

Medicare is funded through the federal (not state) government through general revenues and payroll taxes. Of note, beneficiaries only contribute 13% of the funding through their premiums.[17] Since 1965, costs have far exceeded what beneficiaries have contributed in taxes. For instance, a single man turning 65 in 2010 will receive an average of $180,000 in lifetime Medicare benefits, after contributing $61,000 in lifetime Medicare taxes.[18]

Medicaid

Medicaid is a joint federal–state program established in 1965 to insure the poor. Eligibility and reimbursement policies vary by state, unlike Medicare.

▶ **Eligibility**

These criteria are a little more complicated than those for Medicare. To be eligible, a person must belong to one of the following "categorically eligible" groups:

  ▶ Parents with dependent children
  ▶ Pregnant women
  ▶ People with severe disabilities
  ▶ Seniors (meaning that many Medicaid recipients are "dual eligibles"; that is, they receive both Medicare and Medicaid)
  ▶ Children

States must cover citizens in these groups who have incomes below thresholds based on the federal poverty level (FPL), and there are no enrollment limits—if a state happens to have an unusually high number of residents who fit in these groups, the state must cover them all. States have always had the authority to allow eligibility at higher incomes, and many did, such as Massachusetts.

To make things even more complicated, the ACA mandated a large expansion of Medicaid by declaring that any citizen with an income of 138% or less of the FPL could be enrolled.[e] However, the Supreme Court struck down this part of the law, leaving Medicaid expansion up to individual states. See Chapter 5 for more information on this process—because it has significant and wide-ranging effects. Here we will just say that many states chose not to expand Medicaid and will maintain their prior eligibility criteria, which will lead to big differences in Medicaid coverage and the number of beneficiaries by state.

▶ **Coverage**

Medicaid programs are required to offer minimum benefits, though some states choose to offer more. Required coverage includes:

  ▶ Inpatient and outpatient hospital services
  ▶ Physician, midwife, and nurse practitioner services
  ▶ Laboratory and X-ray services
  ▶ Nursing facility services and home health care for individuals age 21 or older

e   Thus including many low-income adults without dependent children who previously could not get any sort of insurance.

- ▸ Early and periodic screening, diagnosis, and treatment for children under age 21
- ▸ Family planning services and supplies
- ▸ Rural health clinic and federally qualified health center services
▸ **Funding**
Unlike Medicare, which is entirely federally funded, Medicaid is funded by both the federal and state governments.

CHIP

CHIP (sometimes referred to as S-CHIP, for State Children's Insurance Program) is a joint federal–state program established in 1997 to insure low-income children.

▸ **Eligibility**
Low-income children are often covered by Medicaid. At a minimum, Medicaid requires coverage of children up to age six with family incomes less than 138% FPL and up to age 18 with family incomes of or less than 100% FPL. (States may choose to cover children at higher family incomes.)
CHIP's purpose is to expand insurance to children who aren't eligible for Medicaid coverage. However, there are no hard-and-fast rules for eligibility; states have broad authority to set their own rules. As of June 2013, Medicaid covered about 28 million children in the nation, CHIP covered 5.7 million, and seven million children were uninsured.[20]

▸ **Coverage**
Coverage varies by state, and benefits are similar to those under Medicaid. States are allowed to limit coverage below the thresholds for Medicaid, and, further, they may require premiums and deductibles on a sliding scale based on family income level.

▸ **Funding**
CHIP is funded by both the federal and state governments, but federal money makes up a larger percentage of the total funding than it does with Medicaid.[21]

Other Government Insurance

The federal government also insures and delivers care to active duty and retired military personnel:

- ▸ **Veterans Health Administration:** A component of the U.S. Department of Veterans Affairs (VA) that provides medical care to veterans and their families at low or no cost. The VA operates numerous outpatient clinics, hospitals, and long-term health care facilities.

▸ **TRICARE:** A Department of Defense program that provides care to the dependents of active-duty military members and to military retirees and their dependents.

INDIVIDUALLY, ON THE MARKET

Millions of Americans can't obtain insurance through their employers or the government—think of the unemployed, self-employed, early retirees, and those working for companies that don't offer ESI—and must turn to the individual market for coverage. The cost of insurance in this market has almost always been more expensive (for various reasons, but clearly one of those is that there is no employer to defray the cost). Historically, it's been nearly impossible to get insurance through the individual market if you had any pre-existing conditions. So not only was it hard to find coverage in the first place—that coverage was often prohibitively expensive. No wonder few people have been covered by the individual market.

The Affordable Care Act changes this equation by (a) organizing individual insurance through the Marketplaces, (b) disallowing pre-existing conditions as a reason either to deny coverage or to raise premiums, and (c) offering subsidies to purchase insurance through the Exchanges for those making 400% or less of the Federal Poverty Level. The goal is to make the individual market more affordable and easier to navigate. See Chapter 5 for more information. (There's a lot of it!)

NO INSURANCE

We would be remiss in discussing the ways people get insurance if we didn't also talk about those who *don't* get insurance. As of 2010, when the Affordable Care Act passed, the uninsured numbered 47 million, which is more than 15% of the U.S. population.[22] Obviously, one of the big selling points of the Affordable Care Act is that it reduces the number of uninsured. Still, projections post-2014 estimate that 31 million will still be uninsured.[23] These numbers will be higher in states that are choosing not to expand Medicaid. (See Chapter 5 for more about these issues.)

One other category you'll need to know about is the "underinsured"—individuals who do have some health insurance coverage, but not enough to adequately cover their medical expenses; for instance, prescription drugs might not be covered.[19] Calculating the total number of underinsured Americans isn't easy, but one well-accepted 2007 study pegged it at 25 million, a 60% increase since 2003.[24]

Reimbursement Types

Insurers negotiate contracts with individual health care facilities as well as with providers. These contracts may include any of the following reimbursement systems, or even multiple ones (e.g., different rates for outpatient vs. inpatient services).

Payment Models

Each of these forms of reimbursement generates a set fee.

For the physician
- Based on services rendered: Fee-for-Service (FFS)
- Based on another criteria, regardless of services rendered:
  - Per diagnosis: Bundled payments for an "Episode of Illness"
  - Per patient: Capitation
  - Per year: Salary

For the hospital
- Based on services rendered: FFS
- Based on other criteria, regardless of services rendered:
  - Per day: Per Diem
  - Per diagnosis: Bundled payments for an "Episode of Illness"
  - Per patient: Capitation
  - Per year: Global budget

As you might imagine, each reimbursement system has pros and cons, and each creates incentives and influences provider behavior, even if only unconsciously. For instance, if you're getting paid FFS, then you have an incentive to increase the number of services you provide, or to focus on the types of services that get paid the most. (In addition, you're paid by how *much* you do, not how *well* you did it or if you helped the patient.) If you are getting paid per diagnosis or by capitation, you have an incentive to reduce the number of services you provide, since you make more profit the less you spend.

Historically, physicians were paid mostly FFS, but there was—and continues to be—a lot of heated debate. Physicians are mixed on the matter; they often complain about an abdominal MRI scan getting reimbursed $500 whereas doing a physical exam and talking to a patient for half an hour (that is, the art of medicine) might get reimbursed $75. Many pilot programs are testing new payment models, but FFS is still the dominant model at this time.

As stated above, any type of reimbursement has pros and cons and will influence behavior—and thus health outcomes. No system can be perfect, so the question is how to design a system of payment that produces the best health outcomes. Typically, the discussion focuses on paying for *value*, but it is incredibly difficult to define value in health care, and it's tricky to think of what measure denotes value. For instance, if you pay more to physicians who keep their patients out of the hospital, physicians may avoid the sickest patients who are most likely to be hospitalized.

PAY FOR PERFORMANCE AND VALUE-BASED PURCHASING

One more payment system you should know about is Pay For Performance (P4P). P4P has become increasingly popular over the past 10 years as a method of simultaneous quality improvement and cost control. (The term of interest is "value," which takes into account both quality and cost.) P4P is not one single form of reimbursement, and there's a lot of variation among P4P systems in the specific measures used, and how those measures are converted to dollars. Yet all types of P4P plans reimburse based on measures of clinical quality, safety, efficiency, and patient satisfaction; the idea is to incentivize value rather than volume.[25]

P4P is often combined with other reimbursement systems; for example, a single provider might receive 70% of his or her compensation via fee-for-service and 30% from his or her performance on quality measures (e.g., percentage of female patients receiving mammograms), and patient satisfaction.

P4P plays a role in the Affordable Care Act through Value-Based Purchasing (VBP) for hospitals and providers. VBP involves both a quality reporting system and a payment modifier, penalizing those providing below-average care and providing bonuses to those providing above-average care. There are two types of VBP:

▸ The **Hospital VBP** program began in 2012. The Hospital Inpatient Quality Reporting program includes information from 3,500 hospitals. Then hospitals are scored on three measures[26]—how closely hospitals adhered to clinical guidelines for certain diagnoses, how patients scored the care they received, and mortality rates for certain diagnoses. Then, depending on their score, Medicare applies an adjustment factor. Hospitals may lose or gain 1% of payments (which will increase to 2% by 2017).[27]

▸ The **Physician Feedback/Value-Based Payment Modifier** program began rolling out in 2013 and applies to all Medicare providers as of 2017. Previously, only one-third of physicians engaged with the Physician Quality Reporting System;[28] however, the new program requires reporting by all 600,000 providers who bill Medicare. As with the Hospital VBP, providers stand to gain or lose 1% of their payments (increasing to 2% as of 2017). Note, however, that critics fear that the current scoring system is overly focused on primary care and that more evidence is necessary to understand what types of incentives will work with providers.[28]

Of course, it's not so easy. There are strong criticisms of P4P in general and VBP in particular. One criticism is that it is notoriously difficult to measure quality, and VBP has not solved this issue. Further, measuring outcomes without adjusting for context could end up penalizing hospitals that serve poorer, sicker populations—i.e., the hospitals that need resources the most.[29] VBP in particular may complicate matters by "layering" on top of a flawed fee-for-service reimbursement structure.[30] And, in fact, current research shows "modest or inconsistent effectiveness" in attempts by P4P to increase quality.[31] Thus, some worry that P4P means Medicare will effectively be paying for cheaper care without safeguarding quality.[30]

While P4P and VBP are the trend and may ultimately be effective, there are many kinks—in measurement, in designing effective incentives—to be worked out along the way.

How Fees Are Determined

We've gone over some models of payment, which pay a set fee for certain criteria. Now let's look at how those fees get set in the first place, using Medicare fees as an example.

DIAGNOSIS-RELATED GROUP (DRG)

For inpatient care, Medicare pays a flat rate based on the patient's diagnosis.[f,g] DRGs were instituted by Medicare in the early 1980s as a way to reduce costs—they were revolutionary: DRGs shifted reimbursement from *retrospective* to *prospective* payment, and, as the Department of Health & Human Services puts it, "in this DRG prospective payment system, Medicare pays hospitals a flat rate per case for inpatient hospital care so that efficient hospitals are rewarded for their efficiency and inefficient hospitals have an incentive to become more efficient."[32] The DRG payment system has had a huge influence on providers and hospitals, including a significant reduction in average hospital length of stay for patients.[h]

RELATIVE VALUE UNIT

The corresponding system for physicians is known as the relative value unit (RVU). This is a point system that Medicare uses to set reimbursement rates for medical diagnoses, treatments, and procedures under a fee-for-service payment system. Each action a physician undertakes is rated on three factors:

- ▸ Work of the physician (about 50%)
- ▸ Expense to the practice (about 45%)
- ▸ Cost of malpractice insurance (about 5%)[33]

For example, a diagnostic colonoscopy is worth about 6 RVUs, while surgically removing part of the colon is nearly 40 RVUs.[34] The RVU value is multiplied by a conversion factor to determine the amount of money the physician receives for the service.

Remember, while DRGs and RVUs determine payment for services, they have no control over what types of services are offered, nor how often.

---

f   Diagnoses, diseases, symptoms, and the like are all classified according to a mind-numbing system known as the International Classification of Diseases (ICD). The U.S. is currently transitioning between the 9th version of the ICD to the 10th, which will include 140,000 codes, including gems like V9542XA—"Forced landing of spacecraft injuring occupant."

g   Medicare does make allowances for cases that are unusually complicated and expensive. These "outlier cases" are billed separately and at a higher reimbursement rate than a typical DRG.

h   This shift to shorter hospital stays has pros and cons. Though many patients may be glad not to spend the night in a hospital, discharging patients before they're ready has negative consequences both for health (due to incomplete care) as well as for costs (through readmissions and avoidable health outcomes). On the other hand, keeping patients in the hospital for too long puts them at increased risk for hospital-acquired infections and medical errors, and each extra day in the hospital can cost $10,000 or more. For now, though, the drive to reduce length of stay shows no signs of stopping.

AMA/Specialty Society
Relative Value Scale Update Committee (RUC)

Since the early 1990s, the American Medical Association (a professional organization and lobbying group) has operated the RUC, the committee that sets RVUs. The committee comprises 31 physicians, 21 of whom are nominated by specialty societies, representing the array of specialties. The committee polls hundreds of physicians to determine the "time and intensity" required for physicians' work. Once the committee determines RVUs (of which there are thousands), Medicare may choose to adopt the recommendations; in practice, the committee's recommendations are almost always adopted.[35] Medicare then independently sets the price paid per RVU by applying a "conversion factor." For instance, the conversion factor has previously been used to keep reimbursements the same even when RVUs rose.[36]

While RVUs are set for Medicare alone, other insurers use them as well, though they, too, can set whatever price they want per point. As such, the RUC holds quite a bit of power over reimbursement rates for physicians, making it controversial. Here are some of the arguments both critics and supporters make:

Critics	Supporters
▸ The RUC over-represents specialties; only five committee members represent primary care.[37] The committee then overvalues specialty procedures, skewing salaries to the detriment of primary care.	▸ The RUC does support primary care, notably by recommending RVUs for services some primary care physicians provided free of charge. Such support has been undermined by Medicare itself, as well as private payors.[38]
▸ It makes no sense for physicians to set their own reimbursement rates.	▸ Physicians can provide the best information about how to value their work. In addition, the RUC makes recommendations rather than law.
▸ The RUC is too secretive, since those who attend the meetings must sign non-disclosure agreements.[35]	▸ The committee allows members of the public to attend; non-disclosure agreements are to prevent market speculation. In addition, the committee recently voted to publish the dates and times of their meetings, as well as the minutes.[39]

MEDICARE SUSTAINABLE GROWTH RATE

The Medicare Sustainable Growth Rate (SGR) is a method for determining physician reimbursement, in use since 1997. The idea behind the SGR is to make sure that physician payments don't rise faster than the economy in general. The SGR is determined by:[40]

- ▸ Change in physician fees
- ▸ Change in number of Medicare beneficiaries in the fee-for-service program
- ▸ Change in GDP
- ▸ Change in expenditures due to new laws and regulations

Health care costs, though, have been rising much faster than GDP, meaning that each year, the SGR *should* require physician payments to be cut—instead, each year since 1997, Congress has voted to override the SGR and not adjust physician payments. This is called the "doc fix." If, some year, Congress decides not to override the scheduled cuts, then *all* prior cuts will come into effect. For instance, in 2013, physician payments would have been cut by 26.5%.[41] You can imagine how that would have gone over.

Obviously, sidestepping the law every year isn't the best long-term solution. The SGR is pretty unpopular on all sides, and the goal is to create a "permanent doc fix," which will rein in physician payments without the SGR. The various political and professional groups have so far been unable to agree on a replacement plan. (Quite shocking, we know.)

Now that we've looked at what insurance is and how it's administered, let's look at how much U.S. health care costs and then move to the REALLY big question . . . *why* does it cost so much?

How Much Does U.S. Health Care Cost?

In 2012, national health expenditures reached $2.8 trillion, which is $8,915 per person and 17.2% of the nation's gross domestic product (GDP), far more than any other developed country. CMS expects spending to grow by around 6% per year, reaching 19.9% of GDP by 2022.[42] Per capita spending varies widely by state, from $5,031 in Utah to $9,278 in Massachusetts. (For more on regional variation, see Chapter 5.)[42]

Where Health Care Dollars Come From . . .

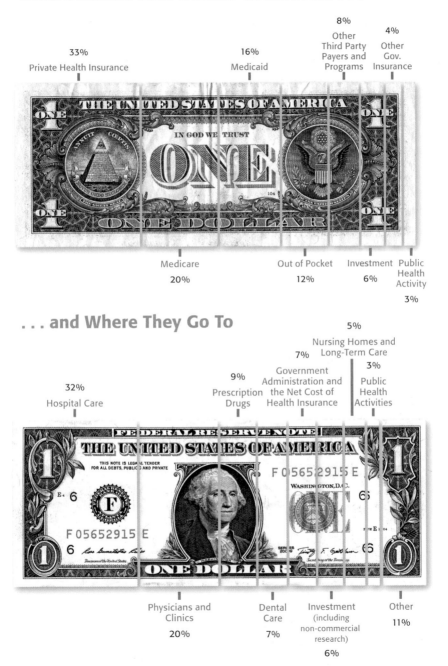

33%
Private Health Insurance

16%
Medicaid

8%
Other Third Party Payers and Programs

4%
Other Gov. Insurance

Medicare
20%

Out of Pocket
12%

Investment
6%

Public Health Activity
3%

. . . and Where They Go To

32%
Hospital Care

9%
Prescription Drugs

7%
Government Administration and the Net Cost of Health Insurance

5%
Nursing Homes and Long-Term Care

3%
Public Health Activities

Physicians and Clinics
20%

Dental Care
7%

Investment (including non-commercial research)
6%

Other
11%

Centers for Medicare & Medicaid Services, "Nation's Health Dollar—Where It Came From, Where It Went," Jan. 2014. Note: Sum of pieces may not equal 100% due to rounding.

An Important Disclaimer: Cost Does Not Equal Price

In health care, the relationship between price (the ability to charge a certain amount for a product) and cost (how much it costs you to produce it) is rarely clear. As the Robert Wood Johnson Foundation puts it, "Little is known about how prices are derived. The answer to the basic question of what health care costs often is unknown. Payers see a bill, but generally are given very little detail about how prices in that bill are determined."[43] To underscore this point, we can look at the fact that different payors pay different amounts for the same services. Keep this in mind when reading about health care costs, prices, charges, and expenditures. Are we talking about the cost or the price? How would the difference matter in that situation?

Distribution of Spending

Distribution of Health Expenditures for the U.S. Population

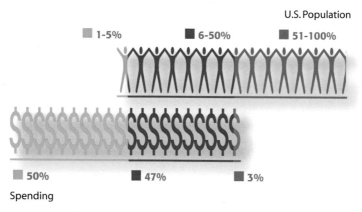

Agency for Healthcare Research and Quality, "Differentials in the Concentration in the Level of Health Expenditures Across Population Subgroups in the U.S., 2010," August 2013.

When analyzing the cost of U.S. health care, it's important to remember that spending is not spread evenly among all patients. According to the Agency for Healthcare Research and Quality, in 2009, 21.8% of health care spending came from just 1% of patients. That's roughly three million people in the U.S. who each spent about $90,000 in a year on health-related expenses. Further, the AHRQ states, "[T]he top decile of spenders were more likely to be in fair or poor health, elderly, female, non-Hispanic whites and those with public-only coverage. Those who remained in the bottom half of spenders were more likely to be in excellent health, children and young adults, men, Hispanics, and the uninsured."[44]

The fact that so many resources go to so few patients led to the term "super-utilizers." Increasingly, policy efforts focus on how to reduce costs among this group.

Health Spending Slowdown

Health care spending has become a bigger and bigger portion of the GDP, rapidly approaching an unsustainable level. Health care spending grew faster than the economy for many years, and that growth hurt. As Jonathan Cohn puts it, "when national health care spending rises much more quickly than the economy is growing, you feel the impact—as relatively higher insurance premiums, higher out-of-pocket costs, and higher taxes to support government insurance programs."[45] For several years, though, the rate at which health spending outpaced the economy has been slowing. That is, overall spending was still growing; it just wasn't accelerating as fast as it was before.

Annual Growth Rates for Health Spending and GDP

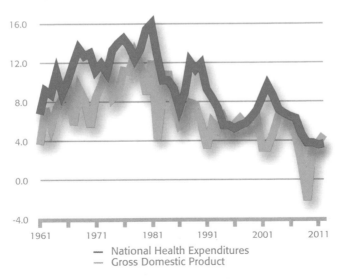

— National Health Expenditures
— Gross Domestic Product

Centers for Medicare & Medicaid Services, "National Health Expenditure Data," Jan. 2014.

Why the slowdown? The Congressional Budget Office (CBO) suggests that Medicare and Medicaid spending slowed in such a breadth of programs that it must be attributed to many factors and that it must include a change in "the behavior of beneficiaries and providers."[46] The big question was whether the causes were temporary (like the recession) or lasting (that is, structural changes that would slow spending growth for the long-term).[47]

The CBO predicted that the slowdown would continue even as the Affordable Care Act was implemented, but others thought the ACA would contribute to higher spending because of increased utilization.[48] As of publication, it was looking like the naysayers might have been right, as spending accelerated again to 6.7%, the highest it had been since the slowdown began in 2007.[49] Does this mean that the slowdown is over, and that costs will rise precipitously again? Not necessarily. But this is certainly an issue to watch.

Why Does U.S. Health Care Cost So Much?

This question has a lot of answers.[i] We've broken the reasons into two categories:
1. Reasons arising from the health care system itself
2. Reasons arising from the nature of disease and of society

After considering those reasons, we will discuss the consequences of high costs and why health care does not function like a "normal" market.

The System Itself

INSURANCE AS INSULATION

Insurance is designed to protect against large, unexpected costs. However, when this protection is too great, or when it covers even relatively small, predictable costs, insurance becomes "insulation," something that protects consumers from the full brunt of the very large cost of health care. Only a tenth of health care spending is currently out-of-pocket, down from nearly 50% in 1960.[22] Many economists claim insulation from prices leads to increased health care spending because people tend to be more cavalier with money when they know they won't be paying the bill—i.e., no one washes a rental car. In addition, health insurance has evolved over time to

---

i   Unfortunately, it's not simply "Because the health care system is so good"—see the Introduction for more.

be considered a right rather than a privilege. When discussing health insurance, it's never simply an economic matter; it also involves values.

LACK OF TRANSPARENCY

For Medicare and other insurers, total health care costs are at least slightly transparent—since they have to reimburse these costs—and they're able to take cost into account when deciding what treatments to cover. No such transparency exists for individual patients, though. Individuals are often asked to account for costs in their medical decision-making; however, many barriers stand in their way:

- Hospitals and physicians don't provide up-front information about prices and billing.
- Patients haven't had access to national data or average costs at individual hospitals.[j]
- Even if patients could access the above data, they would need to compare costs at all regional hospitals and be willing to switch hospitals even if they are in critical condition.
- Patients have no way of knowing whether *their own care* would be comparable. (Their illness may be more severe, they may have more or fewer co-morbidities, their care may have more or fewer complications, etc.).
- Patients usually don't understand how medical billing works.
- Patients usually don't have time to hassle with billing forms and learn about coverage rules.
- Patients lack the clinical knowledge in comparing the added value of a more expensive treatment.

The fact is not just that medical costs aren't transparent—it's also that costs **can never be** fully transparent. Patients have no idea what their care is going to end up costing, and thus their ability to make cost-based decisions is inherently compromised.

LACK OF STANDARDIZATION

The more diversity that exists in payment forms, systems, rules, and payors themselves, the more work time must be devoted to billing. This billing workforce cost has played a role in the decreasing ability of physicians to

---

j   There is now some ability to compare costs here: www.opscost.com/

maintain private practices.[k] Each health care facility must pay for its own dedicated billing department or pay to outsource it (unlike, say, in England, where billing is a centralized organization). Further, each billing department must master different forms and reimbursement rules for each of many different insurers and plans.

In fact, in 2011, research found that "US nursing staff, including medical assistants, spent 20.6 hours per physician per week interacting with health plans," costing $82,975 per physician annually.[50]

And this is just looking at billing! You can just imagine the other ways in which a similar lack of standardization in other departments increases costs.

LACK OF COORDINATION

The U.S. system is decentralized and complicated, with many different organizations providing different aspects of care. Only rarely are these connected

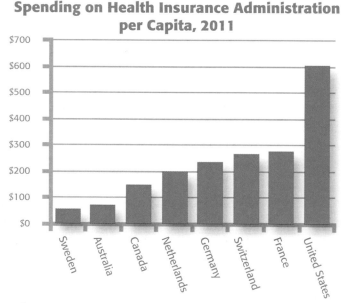

Spending on Health Insurance Administration per Capita, 2011

The Commonwealth Fund, "2013 International Health Policy Survey in Eleven Countries," Nov. 2013. Used with permission. Note: In U.S. $, adjusted for differences in cost of living.

k   Many offices and hospitals outsource their billing services to a specialized business, like the Medical Billing Service, and, as is a trend in other areas of health care, some of this outsourcing is going abroad in an attempt to reduce costs. Interestingly, privacy concerns have both increased billing needs (by increasing the amount of paperwork required by law) and constrained cost-reduction (by raising concerns about privacy in outsourcing).

to one another, and a patient may end up receiving care from multiple organizations without their working to coordinate her or his care. For instance, a patient getting discharged from X hospital may then need home health help from Y home aides, as well as follow-up appointments with Z primary care office. Those transitions provide a lot of opportunities for things to fall through the cracks, so it shouldn't come as a surprise that following hospital discharge nearly half of hospitalized patients experience at least one medical error in medication continuity, diagnostic workup, or test follow-up.[51]

Many of these errors lead to hospital readmissions (and an estimated $12 billion in preventable spending[52]), which has been a major focus of reform efforts. The government cannot force different organizations, like X, Y, and Z above, to coordinate their care, but it *can* penalize hospitals for readmissions—in fact, this is an important part of the Affordable Care Act (see Chapter 1 for more information). The idea is that, if we can incentivize coordination, then we can reduce wasteful spending (while providing a better quality of care).

OVERTREATMENT

Overtreatment occurs when patients receive treatments or procedures that aren't medically necessary. As you might imagine, this raises costs. In 2009, Atul Gawande popularized this issue in a much-discussed article in *The New Yorker.*[53] The idea behind overtreatment is just that: Providers may order—and patients may demand—more expensive tests and procedures than are necessary, and they may diagnose and treat diseases that either aren't there or don't really need *treatment*, per se.

Since newer, more complex tests, procedures, and drugs are expensive, and since health care dollars are limited, it's legitimate to ask how much quality improvement is worth how much cost. Might you, as a patient who suspects abdominal obstruction, be willing to have a $300 X-ray instead of an $1,800 CT scan if the CT scan is only 3% more sensitive? Most patients wouldn't know what the range of diagnoses might be or how to evaluate such a calculation.

They might be likely to either:
▸ Reflexively go with the cheaper one (if paying out-of-pocket) or
▸ Reflexively go with the most state-of-the-art (if insured).

Physicians, who know both the range of diagnoses as well as the benefits of different diagnostics, may be best suited to make the decision, but they, too:

▸ May not be up-to-date on evidence or
▸ May reflexively go with the state-of-the-art imaging if they know their patient is insured.

Policymakers could set a particular cost–benefit calculation for these decisions (as England does), but this may fail to account for outliers (those whose bodies and experiences don't fit the average) and patient choice.

Another difficult issue with overtreatment is physician conflict of interest. Let's say you're a gastroenterologist in a private practice. Because you send so many patients for CT scans, you decide that it would be more efficient to buy a scanner yourself for the office. This may be more convenient for both you and the patient, but it also means that you are now the person who both decides when a patient uses the CT *and* the person who benefits monetarily when they do. Even if you have nothing but the best intentions, this is an obvious conflict of interest.[l]

In an effort to counteract overtreatment by reducing the use of "low value" services, the American Board of Internal Medicine started the Choosing Wisely Campaign in 2012. Choosing Wisely publishes lists of "Five Things Patients and Physicians Should Question" in more than 40 specialties, aiming to "spark discussion" between patients and providers about what tests and treatments to use.[54] For example, the American College of Radiology recommends, "Don't do imaging for uncomplicated headache." The ultimate aim is both to lower costs and to improve quality; the campaign has had excellent buy-in from providers and specialty societies.[m] You can view Choosing Wisely as a sort of grassroots effort by professionals to improve the value of the care they provide, as opposed to policies determined by non-physician lawmakers. That is a remarkable trend, although the impact of the campaign remains to be seen.

---

l   Regulating this conflict of interest faces powerful opposition. First, while the conflict of interest is clear in the hypothetical, physicians may be offended at the thought that their decision-making capabilities could be compromised and, therefore, may oppose attempts at regulation. In addition, manufacturers benefit monetarily when physicians buy separate equipment instead of sharing them and may further oppose attempts at regulation. Thus, both authority and money bolster the status quo.

m   On the other hand, most specialty societies generally named other specialties' services as low-value.

LOOSE GOVERNMENTAL REGULATIONS

Governments in Japan, Germany, and England strictly regulate payments in health care. For instance, in Japan, the government decides what physicians may charge for any service. In Germany, physicians go to school for free but then are salaried. In England, the government negotiates down the price of pharmaceuticals.

Certainly, the U.S. government regulates the health care industry on cost, access, and quality. But our checks on costs are nowhere near those of other industrialized nations. Whether this relative weakness of regulation is good or bad (and there are strong arguments on both sides), it does contribute to higher costs for patients in the U.S.

HIGH PHYSICIAN WAGES

Let's face it: Physicians in the U.S. make a lot of money. In 2012, the median income was $51,017 for all U.S. workers,[55] but $220,942 for primary care physicians and $396,233 for specialists.[56] Those high incomes are reflected in high health care costs.

Obviously, you can offer many reasons why physicians' wages are and should be high (they have incredible responsibility to never make mistakes, they work long hours, their jobs are important to society, they spend many years in training for little or no pay, they have a lot of debt to pay off, etc.), but let's focus on the economic, market-based explanation: Physician supply is limited.

Limited competition contributes to high physician wages, and high physician wages drive up health care costs.

And yet . . . it's not that simple. Areas of the U.S. with the most physicians per capita actually have higher health care spending than average[57] (and the quality isn't any better either).[58] While economic principles tell us that competition should drive costs down, the facts indicate that other factors, like supply-induced demand and overtreatment, may be more powerful in this case. Just another reminder that, when it comes to health care, it's always more complicated than it first appears.

ITERATIVE REIMBURSEMENTS

A large insurer like Blue Cross/Blue Shield gets billed a lot of money by any given hospital, and paying that much means the insurer has leverage (because the hospital needs its payment). The insurers use this leverage when negotiating contracts with hospitals; typically, the insurers only reimburse a percentage of the bill charged by the hospital. This gives hospitals an incentive to simply increase the prices of their services, thereby increasing the amount, if not the percentage, they get reimbursed. The ugly underbelly of this tug of war is that patients who are uninsured or underinsured (that is, those who must pay out-of-pocket) get handed a bill much higher than any insurer would ever actually pay. This undiscounted bill is known in the industry as the "rack rate."

PHARMACEUTICALS AND TECHNOLOGY

Research, development, marketing, and use of new drugs and devices account for a large and growing share of U.S. health care spending. See Chapter 4 for more information about these industries and their financial impact.

EMERGENCY DEPARTMENT OVERUSE

Emergency Departments (EDs) are vital for hospitals since they serve as a major point of entry for inpatients. However, the sheer volume of patients choosing to go to the ED for care when they really should be going to their primary care doctor or to an urgent care center has driven up costs, impeded access, and ultimately affected quality, as well.

In the late 1980s, as health care costs and levels of uninsured patients were growing, concerns arose about EDs turning away patients who couldn't afford care. To combat this, Congress passed the Emergency Medical Treatment and Active Labor Act (EMTALA) in 1986 for all Medicare-participating hospitals (essentially all of them).[59] EMTALA requires EDs to screen all presenting patients to determine whether they have an emergency condition and stabilize patients who are deemed to have one—regardless of that person's ability to pay for care. Partly as a result, ED visits have increased significantly over the past 20 years.

The groups with the highest ED usage rates are Medicaid recipients, the poor, and the elderly.[60] These groups have higher-than-average rates of

Emergency Department Visits and Emergency Departments in Community Hospitals

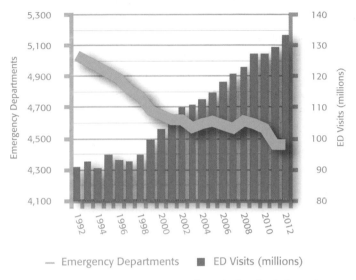

American Hospital Association, "TrendWatch Chartbook," March 2014.
Used with permission.

chronic medical conditions,[61] which often require expensive, ongoing care. And all three groups are more likely to be uninsured[n] or insured by the government. Thus, EDs can be expensive, with a lot of patients who don't pay (although the average hospital still makes enough from insured patients to get about 8% profit from the ED).[62] The average cost of an ED visit in 2011 was $1,354.[63] Fifty-five percent of patients 65 or older receive an X-ray and 29% receive a CT scan during an ED visit.[64]

Solutions proposed to reverse the trend toward overcrowded, costly EDs have been to reduce the utilization of tests and procedures (which some claim is due to defensive medicine) or to increase the availability of community-based outpatient care centers such as urgent care or retail clinics. These centers can attend to medical issues urgent to the patient but not necessary to handle in an ED. The CDC reports, for instance, that one-third of ED visits are semi-urgent or non-urgent and could be handled in other facilities.[64] But some patients continue to go to the ED for care. There may be reasons for this—a patient might rather go to an ED after work than miss work for a PCP appointment, or might

---

n   Note that it is not simply a matter of sending the individual a bill. Many of the uninsured are also impoverished, and they are unable to pay these bills. If such patients do not have wages or assets that a creditor can collect, the hospital will never recoup these costs, even if the patient keeps coming back to the ED.

not have the funds for up-front payment at urgent care. These situations would need to be addressed to change the "culture of the ED."

Disease and Society

CHRONIC DISEASE CARE

Once upon a time, humans died mostly from infectious diseases, but then the advent of sanitation, refrigeration, and vaccination put a damper on such mortality and morbidity. In industrialized nations, at least, the bugs have moved to the back of the bus, leaving room for chronic conditions to step forward. Diabetes, heart disease, high blood pressure, and cancer are ongoing, very expensive chronic conditions that plague the U.S. now, and there is no vaccine or quick cure for them. Diabetes may not be as deadly as smallpox, but it's not curable, and it costs more to treat.

Leading Causes of Death[65]	Deaths	Costliest Conditions[63]	Billions
Heart disease	595,444	Heart disease	$91
Cancer	573,855	Cancer	$71
Chronic lung diseases	137,789	Mental disorders	$60
Stroke	129,180	Trauma-related disorders	$67
Accidents	118,043	Osteoarthritis	$56
Alzheimer's	83,308	Hypertension	$47
Diabetes mellitus	68,905	Diabetes mellitus	$46
Kidney diseases	50,472	Chronic lung diseases	$45
Influenza and pneumonia	50,003	Hyperlipidemia	$39
Suicide	37,793	Back problems	$35

In 2011, six out of the top 10 leading causes of death were from chronic diseases (the bold diseases in the table)—and 50% of American adults live with a chronic disease diagnosis.[66] According to the Centers for Disease Control and Prevention (CDC), the best way to deal with chronic diseases is through prevention. This is worth repeating: Most chronic conditions are preventable through healthy eating and living. Thus, unless the U.S. population begins trending toward healthier lifestyles, chronic conditions will continue—and perhaps grow—as a driver of increased health care spending.

END-OF-LIFE CARE

The cost of end-of-life health care greatly outstrips that of any other time; a full quarter of Medicare spending goes to care in the last year of life.[67] Patients, physicians, and families often "pull out all the stops" to treat those near death, even if the tests and procedures have little chance of succeeding. The bioethicist Arthur Caplan states, "What would you do if your mother needed an expensive, painful operation that had only a one in a million chance of saving her? [. . .] Most Americans would say 'do it.' In this country, we are all about hope."[68]

Unfortunately, you rarely know ahead of time that it's your last year of life. It's obvious that death is inevitable, and, in hindsight, it seems odd to spend hundreds of thousands of dollars to extend lives by only a few months. Yet, for patients and their families in the moment, impending death may not feel obvious. Just as inevitable as death is the fact that health care will always be mediated by emotion. Many patients and families seek to pull out all the stops to prolong life. And that's expensive.

UNHEALTHY BEHAVIORS

Maybe you've heard, but Americans aren't the healthiest people around. An astounding 75% of Americans are either overweight or obese (nearly twice as many as 50 years ago),[69] an epidemic that accounts for more than one-tenth of U.S. health spending.[70,71] Similarly, 18% of American adults smoke tobacco,[72] which causes an array of diseases that rack up $157 billion annually.[73] And those who undergo medical treatment don't always do so perfectly: Less than half of all prescriptions are taken as directed, a lack of adherence that is estimated to cause 10% of all hospital admissions.[74]

The point of this section isn't to heap blame on those who smoke, don't exercise enough, or miss a pill every once in a while (and by no means to suggest these are uniquely American failings, either). The point is that personal behavior and lifestyle affect health, and health itself is the major determinant of health care costs. Health care providers can treat illness and injury, screen for disease, and emphasize healthy behaviors, but, short of following patients home to make sure they eat right and work out, there's only so much providers can do.

POVERTY AND RURAL LIVING

The U.S. government defines the federal poverty level (FPL) by family size, as shown in the table on the right with data from 2014.[75] (These thresholds are the same throughout the nation, excluding Alaska and Hawaii, and don't account for cost-of-living variations.) The thresholds are used to determine eligibility for most government welfare programs, including Medicaid.

Household	Income Threshold
1	$11,670
2	$15,730
3	$19,790
4	$23,850

In 2012, 15% of Americans were living in poverty.[76] While poverty may not always directly worsen health or increase health care spending, it does have far-ranging indirect effects. Living in poverty may affect a person's ability to get proper care as a child, leading to poor health later in life. It may affect the ability to get off from work for appointments or to find work that even offers health insurance. It may correlate with education and ability to understand health information. It may affect the ability to afford needed prescriptions or to buy healthy, nutritious food.

You get the idea. These examples and more adversely affect the health of millions, and poor health increases the health care costs needed for treatment. The U.S. health care system feels the effects of poverty in two ways: first, as a health determinant that physicians lack ability to change; second, by swelling the ranks—and increasing the costs—of public insurance programs.

Similar to those living in poverty, those living in rural areas have a decreased ability to access care. Rural areas have fewer physicians per capita, particularly specialists. And as we have seen, lack of access affects health status, which ultimately affects the cost of care.

POOR HEALTH LITERACY

Normally, we think of literacy as the ability to comprehend the written word. Certainly, reading ability affects health literacy, but it's about more than that. A person's knowledge of anatomy (e.g., where the liver is), body functioning (e.g., that the kidneys process urine), and basic medication information (e.g., don't take medicine on an empty stomach) has a huge impact on how he or she approaches both wellness and disease.

Clinical: Low health literacy is quite widespread in society—even PhDs complain about not understanding their physicians—and a large, nation-wide study showed that only 12% of Americans had proficient health literacy.[77] In a world of ever-increasing knowledge, it's understandable that those who don't specialize in medicine might not know much about it; in the world of health care, it's understandable that health professionals might forget what their patients don't know. Thus, encouraging both general patient education and provider "plain speech" are important goals.

Research: Biomedical research gets published in science journals, using standards, statistical analysis, and jargon that leave the lay reader scratching his or her head. Even with good health literacy and plain speaking in appointments, it's unrealistic to expect even the educated patient to know how to evaluate recent medical evidence. Patients must trust that their providers keep up with the literature, and this has implications for shared decision-making.

Health disparities: Disparities arise in both access and quality of health care, and they're influenced by socioeconomic status, gender, sexuality, geography, ethnicity, language, and culture. All of these categories may influence health literacy as well, but it's interesting to note that low reading literacy is the single best predictor of poor health status.[78] In addition, those with chronic diseases are more likely to have limited literacy.[79] It makes sense that people who have trouble reading their medication labels and understanding their physicians might have difficulty managing their diseases, which has implications not just for individual health outcomes, but also for costs and population health.

Misinformation: We live in an era of incredible access to information; however, not all of it is correct. The media can be misleading ("Carrots Will Kill You," then, six months later: "Carrots Are a Superfood"). And the Internet can be both the best and the worst friend a doctor ever had ("Doc, I have a runny nose, and I read on the Internet that might mean I have lupus!"). Obviously the media and Internet can be an enormous help, but sometimes they confuse, too.

Patients may have difficulty understanding not only what their disease process is, or what their provider is instructing them to do, but what their medicines are and how to take them. Poor understanding can have wide-reaching consequences on behavior. We see them in the following ways:

▸ Over-reliance on providers, e.g., never getting a second opinion or always taking recommendations without sharing your own opinion

▸ Under-reliance on providers, e.g., believing Jenny McCarthy about vaccines or using crystals to cure cancer

▸ Mismanagement of health, e.g., eating unhealthily or not using condoms with new sexual partners

▸ Mismanagement of disease, e.g., skipping pills or eating high-sugar foods as a diabetic

▸ Over-prioritizing innovation, e.g., wanting the newest technology, even when it may not be the actual best

▸ Over-prioritizing cost, e.g., not going to the ED even when you really need to because it costs too much.

Consequences of High Costs

Rationing

Health care is a limited resource: There are restrictions on money, on providers, on time, on supplies, and on technology. Unless all world resources are devoted to health care, rationing must exist.

We already do it. That is a fact, so keep it in mind through every debate about rationing. The current U.S. system rations by restricting access based on ability to pay. All potential reform plans include rationing, too—even if they simply preserve the current practice.

Rationing often gets criticized by pundits and politicians as an erosion of our rights, and certainly it feels appalling to prioritize some lives over others. However, as the ethicist Peter Singer notes,[80] for every patient we hear about in Britain who has to wait three months for a hip replacement or cannot get an experimental cancer treatment funded, there's an American who cannot afford a wheelchair or the standard-of-care chemotherapy medication. Every system rations in some way, and each system has pros and cons. To understand health care, you must acknowledge and comprehend the ways that care is rationed and the effects of that rationing.

The real question is how to choose a method of rationing that is most fair and efficient. Different ways to arrange a system of rationing may be:

▸ By how much a given treatment will extend a patient's life[o] (e.g., prioritize expensive, lifesaving measures for the young or otherwise healthy rather than for the elderly or very ill)

▸ By a patient's ability to pay (e.g., high deductibles for patients or low reimbursements for providers)

▸ By first come, first served (e.g., a waiting list, like those for transplants)

▸ By comparative effectiveness (e.g., prioritize treatments that have been proven to work well)

Being Uninsured

A lot of research has been done on the uninsured: who they are, how they access care, how they do or don't pay for it, what the financial impacts are for society, and what the health impacts are for these individuals. An excellent resource is the Kaiser Family Foundation's *The Uninsured: A Primer,*[6] which is published yearly. All of the following facts are taken from that document (which you really should read in full).

Characteristics[81]

▸ 63% of the uninsured are from families with at least one full-time worker. 90% have a family income below 400% of the federal poverty level, or about $62,000 for a two-person household.

▸ Adults age 26–34 have the highest uninsured rate of any age group: 27.4%.

▸ 80% of the uninsured are U.S. citizens. The uninsured population is 45% White, 15% Black, 32% Hispanic, and 5% Asian.

Care Compensation

▸ In 2008, the average uninsured individual incurred $1,686 in health costs (compared to $4,463 for the non-elderly insured).

▸ The uninsured paid for about one-third of this care out of pocket. About 75% of the remaining, uncompensated cost was paid by federal, state, and local funds appropriated for care of the uninsured, which accounts for about 2% of total health care spending.

▸ 60% of uncompensated care costs are incurred by hospitals.

---

o   A commonly used metric is the Quality-Adjusted Life Year (QALY), which adjusts years of life added by the quality of those years. For example, a year of perfect health would rank as 1 QALY as a baseline, while a year of blindness might be 0.5 QALYs.

> Most government dollars are paid indirectly based on the share of uncompensated care each hospital provides.
> ▸ The percentage of all physicians who provide charity care fell from 76% in 1996–97 to 68% in 2004–05.[82]

Health Care Is Not a Normal Market

Economics is neither an exact nor an all-inclusive science. Thus, we cannot present the above economic concepts without discussing the counterpoint, which suggests that traditional market economics falls short when it tries to explain health care.

As an example, let's look at the discrepancy between market goods and health care. In March of 2012, Supreme Court Justice Antonin Scalia compared purchasing health insurance to purchasing broccoli. When you buy groceries, all the costs are known in advance, but that's not the case with health care.

In purchasing health care services (for instance, surgery to remove an inflamed gallbladder), many factors, some of them unpredictable, produce the total cost. How long will you be in the hospital? What other medical conditions do you have? Will you have a difficult recovery? What drugs are you going to need, and for how long? What tests will be run, and how many? A hospital administrator is not going to be able to tell you these things before the fact. Even within the same institution, there's a huge variance in how much the same procedure costs for different individuals.

Further, even if you could know the cost ahead of time, would that change your behavior? Would you decide not to have gallbladder surgery? Would you go to another hospital? If so, would you also want to know about quality measures for your hospital, surgeon, and nurses? (Good luck finding that data.) What trade-off between cost and quality would be acceptable to you? At the clinic or hospital, would you try to figure out which imaging and tests not to do, or would you trust your doctor to know what's best? And what if the services you turned down were preventive, so your costs increased in the long run?

Often, the most costly medical decisions are made by people under time constraints, at a vulnerable and scary time in their lives. Few have the clinical knowledge—or the desire—to challenge what the doctor suggests.

In fact, the health care system differs from a normal market in many ways beyond this example. Here are a few further examples from multiple sources:[83-85]

- **Information asymmetry:** Patients, providers, hospitals, and insurers all know things that the others don't.
- **Insurance as insulation:** Cost-sharing by insurance hides the real cost from consumers.
- **Conflicting interests:** Physicians may act as both an agent for the patient as well as an independent business owner (or, more broadly, as someone who profits from the care they provide).
- **Tax subsidies:** The tax subsidies provided to employers and employees to purchase insurance distort the market.
- **Failure of competition:** The individual nature of insurance plans and hospitals keeps them from truly competing as market goods.
- **Suppliers are either legally or morally required to provide services:** Emergency departments are required to provide supportive care, local or federal government provides care for those who can't afford it, and providers (including both clinicians and hospitals) are limited by professional and legal limitations from withholding care from those who need it.

Our health—and our health care—is subject to forces outside of our control, and it's also an emotionally and psychologically laden subject. You can choose not to buy a pound of mushrooms. You can't choose not to have heart disease or breast cancer, and you can't expect someone with a health issue to make choices based solely on money. On the other hand, the limitations of the market don't mean that market forces can't be useful in forming a better health care system.

References

1. Internal Revenue Service. Health Savings Accounts and Other Tax-Favored Health Plans. www.irs.gov/publications/p969/ar02.html#en_US_2013_publink1000204020. Accessed July 8, 2014.
2. The Henry J. Kaiser Family Foundation. Health Care Costs: A Primer. www.kff.org/insurance/7670.cfm. Accessed June 10, 2014.
3. Centers for Medicare & Medicaid Services. Shining a Light on Health Insurance Rate Increases. www.cms.gov/CCIIO/Resources/Fact-Sheets-and-FAQs/ratereview.html. Accessed July 8, 2014.
4. Iglehart JK. Defining Medical Expenses—an Early Skirmish over Insurance Reforms. *New England Journal of Medicine.* 2010;363(11):999.

5.   Blumenthal D. Employer-Sponsored Health Insurance in the United States—Origins and Implications. *New England Journal of Medicine.* 2006;355(1):82.

6.   The Henry J. Kaiser Family Foundation. The Uninsured: A Primer—Key Facts About Health Insurance on the Eve of Coverage Expansions. kff.org/uninsured/report/the-uninsured-a-primer-key-facts-about-health-insurance-on-the-eve-of-coverage-expansions/. Accessed July 8, 2014.

7.   Crimmel B. Changes in Self-Insured Coverage for Employer-Sponsored Health Insurance: Private Sector, by Firm Size, 2001-2011—Stat412.Pdf. meps.ahrq.gov/data_files/publications/st412/stat412.pdf. Accessed July 8, 2014.

8.   The Henry J. Kaiser Family Foundation. 2013 Employer Health Benefits Survey. kff.org/private-insurance/report/2013-employer-health-benefits/. Accessed July 8, 2014.

9.   The Henry J. Kaiser Family Foundation. 2013 Employer Health Benefits Survey. kff.org/private-insurance/report/2013-employer-health-benefits/. Accessed July 7, 2014.

10. The Henry J. Kaiser Family Foundation. Snapshots: Employer Health Insurance Costs & Worker Compensation February 2011. www.kff.org/insurance/snapshot/Employer-Health-Insurance-Costs-and-Worker-Compensation.cfm. Accessed July 8, 2014.

11. The Henry J. Kaiser Family Foundation. Snapshots: Trends in Employer-Sponsored Health Insurance Offer Rates for Workers in Private Businesses. kff.org/health-costs/issue-brief/snapshots-trends-in-employer-sponsored-health-insurance-offer-rates-for-workers-in-private-businesses/. Accessed July 8, 2014.

12. Gould E. Employer-sponsored health insurance coverage continues to decline in a new decade. www.epi.org/publication/bp353-employer-sponsored-health-insurance-coverage/. Accessed June 10, 2014.

13. Gruber J. End a Health Insurance Subsidy. *The New York Times.* Nov 14, 2010.

14. The Henry J. Kaiser Family Foundation. Health Insurance Coverage of the Total Population. kff.org/other/state-indicator/total-population/. Accessed July 8, 2014.

15. The Henry J. Kaiser Family Foundation. Medicare Advantage Enrollees as a Percent of Total Medicare Population. kff.org/medicare/state-indicator/enrollees-as-a-of-total-medicare-population/. Accessed June 23, 2014.

16. How Medicare Supplement Insurance (Medigap) Policies Work with Medicare Advantage Plans. www.medicare.gov/supplement-other-insurance/medigap/medigap-and-medicare-advantage/medigap-and-medicare-advantage-plans.html. Accessed June 23, 2014.

17. The Henry J. Kaiser Family Foundation. Medicare at a Glance. kff.org/medicare/fact-sheet/medicare-at-a-glance-fact-sheet/. Accessed July 3, 2014.

18. Steuerle E, Quakenbush C. Social Security and Medicare Taxes and Benefits over a Lifetime. www.urban.org/UploadedPDF/412660-Social-Security-and-Medicare-Taxes-and-Benefits-Over-a-Lifetime.pdf. Accessed July 8, 2014.

19. Gold J. The 'Underinsurance' Problem Explained. www.kaiserhealthnews.org/Stories/2009/September/28/underinsured-explainer.aspx. Accessed July 8, 2014.

20. Rudowitz R, Artiga S, Arguello R. Children's Health Coverage: Medicaid, CHIP and the ACA. kff.org/health-reform/issue-brief/childrens-health-coverage-medicaid-chip-and-the-aca/. Accessed July 8, 2014.

21. MACPAC. Federal CHIP Financing. www.gpo.gov/fdsys/pkg/GPO-MACPAC-MACBasics-CHIP-2011-09/pdf/GPO-MACPAC-MACBasics-CHIP-2011-09.pdf. Accessed July 3, 2014.

22. Centers for Medicare & Medicaid Services. National Health Expenditure Data. www.cms.gov/Research-Statistics-Data-and-Systems/Statistics-Trends-and-Reports/NationalHealthExpendData/index.html?redirect=/NationalHealthExpendData/. Accessed July 8, 2014.

23. CBO. Updated Estimates of the Effects of the Insurance Coverage Provisions of the Affordable Care Act. www.cbo.gov/sites/default/files/cbofiles/attachments/45231-ACA_Estimates.pdf. Accessed July 8, 2014.

24. Schoen C, Collins SR, et al. How Many Are Underinsured? Trends among U.S. Adults, 2003 and 2007. *Health Affairs.* 2008;27(4):w298.

25. Rosenthal MB, Dudley RA. Pay-for-Performance. *JAMA: The Journal of the American Medical Association.* 2007;297(7):740.

26. Rau J. Methodology: How Value Based Purchasing Payments Are Calculated. www.kaiserhealthnews.org/stories/2013/november/14/value-based-purchasing-medicare-methodology.aspx. Accessed July 8, 2014.

27. Centers for Medicare & Medicaid Services. FAQ Hospital Value-Based Purchasing Program. www.cms.gov/Medicare/Quality-Initiatives-Patient-Assessment-Instruments/hospital-value-based-purchasing/Downloads/FY-2013-Program-Frequently-Asked-Questions-about-Hospital-VBP-3-9-12.pdf. Accessed June 10, 2014.

28. Chien A, Rosenthal M. Medicare's Physician Value-Based Payment Modifier—Will the Tectonic Shift Create Waves? *New England Journal of Medicine.* Nov 28, 2013 2013(369):2076.

29. The Incidental Economist. Paying for Performance—Great in Theory, Not So Much in Reality. blog.academyhealth.org/paying-for-performance-great-in-theory-not-so-much-in-reality/. Accessed July 8, 2014.

30. Goitein L. The Argument Agaisnt Reimbursing Physicians for Value. *JAMA Internal Medicine.* 2014;174(6):845.

31. Epstein A. Will Pay for Performance Improve Quality of Care? The Answer Is in the Details. *New England Journal of Medicine.* 2012(367):1852.

32. Gottlober P. Medicare Hospital Prospective Payment System: How DRG Rates Are Calculated and Updated. *Office of the Inspector General.* 2001.

33. National Health Policy Forum. Relative Value Units. www.nhpf.org/library/the-basics/Basics_RVUs_02-12-09.pdf. Accessed June 21, 2014.

34. Centers for Medicare & Medicaid Services. Physician Fee Schedule. www.cms.gov/apps/physician-fee-schedule/license-agreement.aspx. Accessed July 8, 2014.

35. Whoriskey P, Keating D. How a Secretive Panel Uses Data That Distorts Doctors' Pay. *The Washington Post.* July 20, 2013.

36. American Medical Association. Fact Sheet: Response to *The Washington Post's* "How a Secretive Panel Uses Data That Distorts Doctors' Pay." www.ama-assn.org/ama/pub/news/news/2013/2013-07-22-washington-post-ruc-fact-sheet.page. Accessed July 9, 2014.

37. Moore K, Felger T, et al. What Every Physician Should Know About the RUC. *Family Practice Management.* 2008;15(2):36.

38. American Medical Association. The American Medical Association/Specialty Society Rvs Update Committee's Long History of Improving Payment for Primary Care Services. www.ama-assn.org/resources/doc/rbrvs/ruc-primary-care.pdf. Accessed July 3, 2014.

39. Whoriskey P. AMA Panel Takes Steps toward More Transparency. *The Washington Post.* Nov. 6, 2013.

40. American Medical Association. Medicare and the Sustainable Growth Rate. www.ama-assn.org/resources/doc/mss/cola_medicare_pres.pdf. Accessed July 3, 2014.

41. Kaiser Health News. Congressional Accord Preserves Medicare Doctor Pay. www.kaiserhealthnews.org/Daily-Reports/2013/January/02/fiscal-cliff-doc-fix-and-CLASS-act.aspx. Accessed July 9, 2014.

42. Centers for Medicare & Medicaid Services. NHE Fact Sheet. www.cms.gov/Research-Statistics-Data-and-Systems/Statistics-Trends-and-Reports/NationalHealthExpendData/NHE-Fact-Sheet.html. Accessed July 8, 2014.

43. Painter M, Chernew, M. Counting Change: Measuring Health Care Prices, Costs, and Spending. www.rwjf.org/en/research-publications/find-rwjf-research/2012/03/counting-change.html. Accessed July 8, 2014.

44. AHRQ. The Concentration and Persistence in the Level of Health Expenditures over Time: Estimates for the U.S. Population, 2009-2010. meps.ahrq.gov/mepsweb/data_files/publications/st392/stat392.shtml. Accessed July 3, 2014.

45. Cohn J. Cause for Concern: Health-Care Costs Are Rising—and the Experts Aren't Sure Why. www.newrepublic.com/article/117452/rising-health-care-costs-what-it-means-economy-obamacare. Accessed July 8, 2014.

46. Elmendorf D. The Slowdown in Health Care Spending. www.cbo.gov/publication/44596. Accessed June 23, 2014.

47. Kliff S. The $2.8 Trillion Question: Are Health Costs Growing Fast Again? www.vox.com/2014/4/15/5612900/health-spending-growth-fast. Accessed July 8, 2014.

48. Liu T. The ACA Did Not Cause the Slowdown in Spending—but It May Be Contributing to the Recent Uptick. theincidentaleconomist.com/wordpress/the-aca-did-not-cause-the-slowdown-in-spending-but-it-may-be-contributing-to-the-recent-uptick-2/. Accessed July 9, 2014.

49. Altarum Institute: Systems Research For Better Health. Health Spending Growth Ramps up to Pre-Recession Levels. altarum.org/about/news-and-events/health-spending-growth-ramps-up-to-pre-recession-levels. Accessed July 9, 2014.

50. Morra D, Nicholson S, et al. US Physician Practices Versus Canadians: Spending Nearly Four Times as Much Money Interacting with Payers. *Health Affairs.* 2011-08-01 2011;30(8):1443.

51. Moore C, Wisnivesky J, et al. Medical Errors Related to Discontinuity of Care from an Inpatient to an Outpatient Setting. *Journal of General Internal Medicine.* 2003;18(8):645.

52. Burton R. Health Policy Brief: Improving Care Transitions. *Health Affairs.* Sept. 13, 2012.

53. Gawande A. The Cost Conundrum. *The New Yorker,* June 2009.

54. American Board of Inernal Medicine. Things Physicians and Patients Should Question. www.choosingwisely.org/doctor-patient-lists/. Accessed July 9, 2014.

55. Hargreaves S. 15% of Americans Living in Poverty. money.cnn.com/2013/09/17/news/economy/poverty-income/index.html. Accessed July 9, 2014.

56. Bureau of Labor Statistics. Physicians and Surgeons: Occupational Outlook Handbook. www.bls.gov/ooh/healthcare/physicians-and-surgeons.htm. Accessed July 3, 2014.

57. Fisher E, Wennberg D, et al. The Implications of Regional Variations in Medicare Spending. Part 1: The Content, Quality, and Accessibility of Care. *Annals of Internal Medicine.* 2003;138(4):273.

58. Goodman DC, Fisher ES. Physician Workforce Crisis? Wrong Diagnosis, Wrong Prescription. *New England Journal of Medicine.* 2008;358(16):1658.

59. American Academy of Emergency Medicine. EMTALA: The Basic Requirements, Recent Court Interpretations, and More HCFA Regulations to Come. Accessed July 8, 2014.

60. Garcia T, Bernstein A, et al. Emergency Department Visitors and Visits: Who Used the Emergency Room in 2007? www.cdc.gov/nchs/data/databriefs/db38.htm#ref1. Accessed July 9, 2014.

61. Newton MF, Keirns CC, et al. Uninsured Adults Presenting to US Emergency Departments. *JAMA: The Journal of the American Medical Association.* 2008;300(16):1914.

62. Wilson M, Cutler D. Emergency Department Profits Are Likely to Continue as the Affordable Care Act Expands Coverage. *Health Affairs.* 2014;33(5):792.

63. Agency for Healthcare Research and Quality. Medical Expenditure Panel Survey. meps.ahrq.gov/mepsweb/index.jsp. Accessed June 19, 2014.

64. National Center for Health Statistics. Health, United States, 2012 with Special Feature on Emergency Care. www.cdc.gov/nchs/data/hus/hus12.pdf. Accessed June 9, 2014.

65. Hoyert D, Xu J. Deaths: Preliminary Data for 2011. *National Center for Health Statistics.* 2012;61(6).

66. Centers for Disease Control and Prevention. Chronic Diseases and Health Promotion. www.cdc.gov/chronicdisease/overview/index.htm. Accessed June 23, 2014.

67. Hogan C, Lunney J, et al. Medicare Beneficiaries' Costs of Care in the Last Year of Life. *Health Affairs.* 2001;20(4):188.

68. Duncan D. What Price for Medical Miracles? High Costs at End of Life Still Part of National Health Debate. www.kaiserhealthnews.org/Stories/2010/March/09/fiscal-times-end-of-life.aspx. Accessed July 9, 2014.

69. Ogden C, Carroll M. Prevalence of Overweight, Obesity, and Extreme Obesity among Adults: United States, Trends 1960-1962 through 2007-2008. www.cdc.gov/NCHS/data/hestat/obesity_adult_07_08/obesity_adult_07_08.pdf. Accessed July 8, 2014.

70. Cawley J, Meyerhoefer C. The Medical Care Costs of Obesity: An Instrumental Variables Approach. *Journal of Health Economics.* 2011.

71. Finkelstein EA, Trogdon JG, et al. Annual Medical Spending Attributable to Obesity: Payer- and Service-Specific Estimates. *Health Affairs.* 2009;28(5):w822.

72. Centers for Disease Control and Prevention. Adult Cigarette Smoking in the United States: Current Estimates. www.cdc.gov/tobacco/data_statistics/fact_sheets/adult_data/cig_smoking/. Accessed July 9, 2014.

73. National Center for Chronic Disease Prevention and Health Promotion, Office on Smoking and Health. *The Health Consequences of Smoking: A Report of the Surgeon General.* Washington, D.C.: U.S. G.P.O.; 2004.

74. Haynes RB, McDonald H, et al. Interventions for Helping Patients to Follow Prescriptions for Medications. *Cochrane database of systematic reviews (Online).* 2002;(2)(2):CD000011.

75. U.S. Department of Health & Human Services. 2014 Poverty Guidelines. aspe.hhs.gov/poverty/14poverty.cfm. Accessed June 10, 2014.

76. United States Census Bureau. Poverty. www.census.gov/hhes/www/poverty/about/overview/index.html. Accessed July 9, 2014.

77. National Center for Education Statistics. National Assessment of Adult Literacy (NAAL) —Health Literacy—Highlights of Findings. nces.ed.gov/naal/health_results.asp. Accessed July 8, 2014.

78. Lagay F. Reducing the Effects of Low Health Literacy. *Virtual Mentor.* 2003;5(6).

79. Office of Disease Prevention and Health Promotion. Quick Guide to Health Literacy. http://www.health.gov/communication/literacy/quickguide/factsliteracy.htm. Accessed July 9, 2014.

80. Singer P. Why We Must Ration Health Care. July 15, 2009. *New York Times.*

81. The Henry J. Kaiser Family Foundation. The Uninsured: A Primer—Tables and Data. kff.org/report-section/the-uninsured-a-primer-2013-tables-and-data-notes/. Accessed July 10, 2014.

82. Cunningham P, May J. A Growing Hole in the Safety Net: Physician Charity Care Declines Again. www.hschange.com/CONTENT/826/. Accessed July 3, 2014.

83. Wells D, Ross J, Detsky A. What Is Different About the Market for Health Care? *JAMA: The Journal of the American Medical Association.* 2007;298(23).

84. Frakt A. Health Care Market Failures (and What Can Be Done About Them). theincidentaleconomist.com/wordpress/health-care-market-failures-and-what-can-be-done-about-them/. Accessed July 10, 2014.

85. Fordham Corporate Law Forum. Healthcare Is Not a Free Market, and Never Will Be. That's Why We Need the Mandate. fordhamcorporatecenter.org/2012/04/01/healthcare-is-not-a-free-market-and-never-will-be-thats-why-we-need-the-mandate/. Accessed July 9, 2014.

Chapter 3
Quality, Technology, and Medical Malpractice

Quality, technology, and medical malpractice may seem like an odd mish-mash of topics, but all three share a theme: to make medicine better. This chapter aims to familiarize the reader with major initiatives to measure and improve health care quality—but also to emphasize what a difficult task that is.

Quality

Improving the quality of health care in the U.S. seems to be the one thing that all parties—patients, providers, private companies, and government— can agree on. However, as in many other areas of health care, quality improvement has proven to be a much tougher nut to crack than many had hoped.

The first problem shows up in defining what quality even is. Perhaps defining what quality is *not* is easier. The Agency for Healthcare Research and Quality (AHRQ) discusses health care quality failures in four categories (with examples for each):

> ▸ **Underuse of services:** Only a third of Americans with heart disease receive the influenza vaccine[1] despite evidence that it significantly decreases risk of heart attack.[2]
>
> ▸ **Overuse of services:** Half of all patients diagnosed with the common cold are incorrectly prescribed antibiotics.[3]
>
> ▸ **Misuse of services:** Up to 18% of hospital admissions may result in harm as a consequence of procedures, medications, hospital-acquired infections, diagnostic procedures, and falls.[4]
>
> ▸ **Variation of services:** Medicare patients in Alabama are 8 times more likely to receive epidural steroid injections for low back pain than are Medicare patients in Hawaii.[5]

In contrast, the AHRQ defines quality as "doing the right thing at the right time in the right way for the right person and having the best results possible."[6] That seems pretty straightforward, but also vague. The real trouble is in *measuring* and *comparing* quality of health care.

The University of Michigan health services researcher Avedis Donabedian developed the "Donabedian Triad" as a framework for measuring quality. The triad has three arms: structure, process, and outcomes, and is widely used throughout the health care industry. The physician Bob Wachter summarizes the Donabedian Triad here:

Measure	Advantages	Disadvantages
STRUCTURE How was care organized?	▸ May be highly relevant in a complex health system ▸ Easiest to measure	▸ May fail to capture the quality of care by individual providers ▸ Difficult to determine a "gold standard"
Example: How many patients is each nurse caring for?		
PROCESS What was done?	▸ More easily measured and acted upon than outcomes ▸ May not require case mix adjustment ▸ No time lag—can be measured when care is provided	▸ A proxy for outcomes ▸ All may not agree on "gold standard" ▸ Could promote "cookbook" medicine; providers and health systems may try to "game" their performance
Example: What percentage of patients was given antibiotics before surgery?		
OUTCOMES What happened to the patient?	▸ This is what we really care about	▸ May take years to occur ▸ May not reflect quality of care ▸ Requires case mix adjustments to account for different patient populations
Example: What percentage of patients are still alive 1 year after heart surgery?		

This debate about measuring and comparing health care quality has increasing importance because real money is at stake. Insurance companies, state and federal government programs are tying payments for health care services to quality measurements, and many quality measurements for hospitals and other facilities are now posted online for patients to check out. This means a lot of focus on identifying the correct quality measures and adjusting them appropriately for differences in patient populations and severity of illness. Below we highlight several major issues related to health care quality, but before we do, let's define some important terms.

"Safety" is basically the first part of the Hippocratic Oath: First, do no harm. Or, as the AHRQ puts it, safety is "freedom from accidental or preventable injuries produced by medical care."[7] An **"adverse event"** is any harm that occurs to a patient because of his or her medical care or stay in a health care institution. An adverse event may occur when a mistake has been made or when best practices were followed, but a bad outcome still resulted, like a patient having an allergic reaction to a new medicine. One recent study found that adverse events occur during one-third of hospital admissions.[8] **"Medical errors"** refer more specifically to *preventable* adverse events that occur due to errors during the delivery of care. Examples include a physician making an incorrect diagnosis, a nurse giving medicines to the wrong patient, an IV pump failing during surgery, and a blood test not being ordered due to miscommunication among hospital staff.

Patient Safety

Medical errors have been a major focus of improving health care quality for the past two decades, especially after *To Err is Human: Building a Safer Health System*[9] was published in 1999 by the Institute of Medicine. The report shed light on medical errors, suggesting that 46,000–98,000[a] people died every year from these errors, more than from Alzheimer's disease or drug overdose.[10] This publication had a huge impact, initiating research about communication, guidelines, and information technology to prevent errors.

The medical errors that loom largest in popular consciousness may be cases in which surgeons have operated on the wrong limb. However, these cases are rare. The most common medical errors aren't due to negligence. Rather, most errors occur because of deficiencies within the incredibly complex health care delivery system. Think of a large hospital—a fast-paced, stressful environment with thousands of employees and a dizzying array of computer systems and medical devices. It's easy to imagine how a small miscommunication or oversight can lead to an unintended event. Efforts to stem medical errors don't simply target errors by providers but often focus on improving health care *system* design and on enhancing the transfer of information between providers. Eliminating human error is impossible; instead, creating a safe system where human errors are anticipated and prevented should be the key. *To Err is Human* suggests that "mistakes can best be prevented by designing the health system at all levels to make it safer—to make it harder for people to do something wrong and easier for them to do it right."[9]

Several governmental and nongovernmental bodies oversee patient safety issues for health institutions. The Affordable Care Act addressed some of the IOM's suggestions about coordination for patient safety by mandating the creation a National Quality Strategy.[11] The Joint Commission releases a

---

a   If that strikes you as an awfully big range, don't worry—you're not the first to notice.

list of National Patient Safety Goals[12] every year, and the National Quality Forum lists 34 Safe Practices for Better Healthcare.[13]

Medication Errors

Medications are amazing: They make people feel better and save lives. Unfortunately, every medication also has risks, including toxicity, side effects, and interactions with other drugs. Thus, medications are an important area of safety concern and a focus of quality improvement. In the hospital, about 5% of patients experience an adverse drug event (ADE) and 10–15% experience a "potential" ADE (meaning that no harm was caused by the error).[14] Out of the hospital, nearly 25% of patients experienced an ADE—leading to 700,000 ER visits and 100,000 hospitalizations each year.[14]

It's not just bad handwriting that leads to medication errors, either. See the chart below—and keep in mind that the "prescribing" stage can include many pitfalls; the "Eight Rights" of medication administration are "right patient, right medication, right dose, right route, right time, right

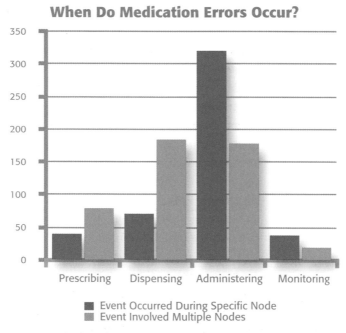

When Do Medication Errors Occur?

■ Event Occurred During Specific Node
■ Event Involved Multiple Nodes

Huber, et al., "ECRI Institute PSO Deep Dive™ Analyzes Medication Events," Sept./Oct. 2012. Used with permission. Note: 695 medication events from 80 health care organizations were analyzed; node was not determined for 25 events.

documentation, right reason, right response."[15] Each of those can and often does become a wrong.

All of these ADEs occur in part because we take so many medications. About 30% of adults take five or more medications,[14] which can get confusing—and there are plenty of other reasons to make a mistake, too. Some of the biggest risk factors for an ADE are age (either very old or very young), a long list of medications ("polypharmacy"), limited health literacy, and especially risky medications (e.g., warfarin, a blood thinner).

Medication errors aren't just dangerous, they're costly. Costs due to medication errors in the U.S. add up to more than $17 billion per year.[16]

Transitions of Care

People get sick 24/7. In an ideal world, a provider who knows the patient would be available anytime, anywhere, for any type of care and would treat the patient until he or she is well again. Unfortunately, physicians and nurses have to sleep, too, so patients will inevitably have their care transferred from provider to provider, nurse to nurse, and system to system. Any time the care of a patient changes hands, there is a risk of necessary information falling through the cracks. The AHRQ compares transitions to a game of telephone—a rather dangerous one, considering that "an estimated 80% of serious medical errors involve miscommunication between caregivers when patients are transferred or handed-off."[17] Here, we will discuss two foci of such transitions: first, transferring care of an inpatient (called a **"handoff"** or "sign out") and, second, transferring a patient from an inpatient setting to the outpatient world (called **"disposition"**).

HANDOFFS

This topic heated up in 2003 when the ACGME (Accreditation Council for Graduate Medical Education) implemented resident work hour restrictions—effectively increasing the number of handoffs. A subsequent study found that any given patient experienced 15 handoffs during a five-day hospitalization, and a resident physician participated in 300 handoffs during a month-long rotation.[18] A good handoff will let the new provider know how sick a patient is, active medical problems and treatments, and issues that might develop. Some of the major problems with improving handoffs are (a) most providers receive little to no education about how to perform handoffs, (b) there is no accepted standard for what handoffs should look like, and (c) most handoffs take place rapidly and in a noisy environment. Different handoff mnemonics have been suggested, such as SBAR, or I-PASS in pediatrics,[19] but none has fully taken root. Research looking at handoff improvements, including standardization, has shown mixed evidence in terms of improving patient outcomes,[20] though a large study in 2013[21] indicated a reduction in medical errors. Regardless, many efforts are being made to improve handoffs. In the meantime, the danger of increased handoffs is the trade-off for reducing work hours.

DISPOSITION

Disposition is the transfer of a patient from one health care setting to another; for instance, a patient who is discharged from the hospital to home with a follow-up appointment to see the primary care doctor within a week. This is a vulnerable time, particularly since so many patients are discharged with new diagnoses and medicines, test results pending, with part of their diagnostic work-up to be completed as an outpatient, and with family members who are expected to provide care without proper—or any—training. Studies have shown that nearly 20% of patients experience an adverse event within three weeks of discharge—the majority of which could have been prevented.[22] Discharge instructions are often given in a rushed manner to patients as they are headed out the door, without ensuring that patients and their families understand and repeat back what they've heard. Repeating back in such a situation is called "closed loop" communication.

The Affordable Care Act intensifies the focus on this issue, and here's why: Poor transfer of care leads to poor health outcomes for patients, which often leads to readmission to a hospital and more expensive care. Up to 20% of Medicare patients are readmitted to the hospital within 30 days of discharge[23]—a high enough number to explain why this is such a priority. CMS began publishing readmission rates for certain conditions in 2009, and the ACA mandates that hospitals will now be penalized for too many of such readmissions. (See "Readmissions Under Reform" in Chapter 1.)

One area of focus is making sure patients leave the hospital on the correct medications, called "medication reconciliation." Health care providers in the hospital often don't have access to patients' outpatient medication lists, and, while hospitalized, a number of medications are started, stopped, and modified. Even in hospitals with advanced electronic systems, keeping track of these medication changes can be tricky. Research has uncovered evidence of discrepancies in medications lists in about one-third of hospital admissions and in 14% of hospital discharges.[24] As you can imagine, patients who are mistakenly taking the wrong medicines will often have poor health outcomes. In 2005, The Joint Commission named medication reconciliation a National Patient Safety Goal, requiring hospitals to implement a standard review process of medications at admission, transfer, and discharge. They have since highlighted these processes when evaluating hospitals, though there is no "gold standard" for medication reconciliation that is used across the nation.

Medication reconciliation is relatively low-hanging fruit for quality improvement; improving the entire transition of care is a lot more difficult, in part because it's clear the process must rely on teamwork among providers and systems that must work together in new ways.

Residency Work Hours

Work hours for resident physicians have long been controversial. Historically, residents lived in the hospital and worked up to 120 hours per week—quite a bit more than the typical 40. Aside from these kinds of hours being difficult psychologically, research shows that overworked, fatigued residents make more mistakes, driving up the medical error rate. Amid such criticism, in 2003, the ACGME limited residency work hours for all programs to 80 per week. In addition, as of July 2011, shifts for first-year residents (also called interns) are limited to 16 hours (second-years and beyond may be scheduled for 28-hour shifts).

Few on either side of the issue consider this to be a satisfactory conclusion, and the debate continues. A few examples of the opposing arguments are outlined in this table.

Point: More Hours Are Better	Counterpoint: Fewer Hours Are Better
▸ The more hours you spend in the hospital, the more you learn; residency is an intense training period by necessity and shouldn't be diluted.	▸ It's inhumane to physicians (psychologically, physiologically, and emotionally) and drives off potential physicians from entering the field.
▸ Patient mortality has not decreased after the institution of the 80-hour work week.[25]	▸ Long work hours encourage more students to enter high-paying specialties so that the money will make up for their time.
▸ Old hours were so long that residents didn't have to rush; now they have to rush constantly and have less time to learn.	▸ Sleep-deprived residents make more errors and decrease patient safety.[26]
▸ Medicine is a career, and training physicians should be completely devoted to it at the expense of other parts of life.	▸ Oversight on residents is weak, meaning many errors will go unnoticed by supervising physicians.
▸ Shorter shifts mean more shift changes, and more handoffs mean more medical errors.[27]	▸ Physicians should value work–life balance.
▸ 80 hours isn't really a limit; residents may work more hours yet only report 80.	▸ We should be seeking to reduce handoff errors in general, not ignoring the problem by increasing shift lengths.
▸ You can't expect to reduce training by 20% without an accompanying reduction in quality.	▸ The U.S. government limits pilots' and truckers' work hours, why not physicians'?

We should note, however, that so far the evidence is mixed on what—if any—effect work hour restrictions have had on patient safety.[28]

Checklists

The idea of a checklist is to standardize, for a particular setting or procedure, a list of things that need to be done (to prevent errors, to prevent infections), then make sure each thing on the list has in fact been done. This sounds deceptively simple but has been shown to have a major impact on quality of care and health outcomes. You may have heard of Atul Gawande's book *The Checklist Manifesto;* the idea of checklists in health care did not originate with Dr. Gawande, but he has popularized the research for the public.

One example of a successful checklist is the Keystone ICU project, which, in 2006, was shown to reduce catheter-related bloodstream infections by 66%.[29] An example of an unsuccessful checklist intervention comes from the city of Ontario, Canada. From 2009 to 2011, Ontario instituted surgical safety checklists at all hospitals, allowing for a population-based study of their effectiveness. The researchers found negligible changes in surgical outcomes.[30]

Checklists are an important experiment for improving quality, and we are likely to see much more research in this vein. They will likely be required in many situations in the future, though proponents point out that, to avoid Ontario's result, checklists shouldn't be used on their own but should be part of a change in team culture (see "Culture Change" later in this chapter).

Never Events

Not all adverse events are preventable, and not all of them are a big deal. It's not fun to feel nauseous after general anesthesia wears off, but it won't ruin your life. Some errors, though, are both catastrophic for patients, and easily preventable. These are called **"never events,"** and the National Quality Forum has identified 29 of them.[31] Medicare and Medicaid have stopped reimbursing hospitals and physicians for any care related to the following never events:

 ▸ Surgery on the wrong body part or wrong patient
 ▸ Wrong surgery on a patient
 ▸ Foreign object left in patient after surgery
 ▸ Death/disability associated with intravascular air embolism, incompatible blood, or hypoglycemia
 ▸ Stage 3 or 4 pressure ulcers after admission
 ▸ Death/disability associated with electric shock, a burn incurred within facility, or a fall within facility[32]

You can see why Medicare wants to stop paying for these occurrences! Despite the terminology, "never events" still happen regularly—for example, more than 300 occur per year in Massachusetts alone.[33]

Health Care-Associated Infections

Health care-associated infections (HAIs), also called nosocomial infections, are diseases that result from hospital treatment; they're infections or conditions that arise *due to* the care patients receive. Obviously, this is the reverse of how things are supposed to be, yet HAIs are all too common. The most recent analysis, from the Centers for Disease Control and Prevention (CDC), estimated that the total number of HAIs for the year 2011 was 721,800 and that about 75,000 patients with HAIs died during their hospitalizations.[34] That means one in 25 hospitalized patients gets an HAI, which are usually more resistant to antibiotics than typical infections and therefore tougher to treat. As if that weren't bad enough, HAIs are also expensive—another CDC report calculated that HAIs cost hospitals between $35 and $45 billion per year.[35] In an effort to improve quality *and* lower costs, Medicare has not reimbursed hospitals for any care related to certain HAIs, including catheter-associated urinary tract infections and surgical site infections after certain elective surgeries,[36] since 2008. Another initiative seeks to make HAIs transparent: Medicare publically reports rates of some HAIs,[b] and many states require hospitals to report their HAI rates. Both payment refusal and transparency are incentives for hospitals to prevent HAIs.

Although it may not be possible to completely eliminate HAIs, many preventive measures have been shown to help—too many for us to cover here. One common example, though, is that proper hand hygiene has been shown to significantly reduce infection rates.[37] But it's worth noting that the CDC guidelines for properly washing hands are two-and-a-half pages long—which may be why researchers estimate that only about 40% of health care workers actually adhere to these guidelines.[38] As with so many issues in health care, behavior change is both absolutely necessary and incredibly difficult.

Importance of Nursing

Nurses are usually the providers who have the most direct contact with patients, and they actually perform the bulk of the care: placing IVs, administering medications, diagnosing pressure ulcers, placing urinary catheters, monitoring vital signs, putting patients on fall risk precautions—the list

---

b   You can check them out for yourself at HospitalCompare.hhs.gov

goes on. As you might imagine, then, nursing has an enormous impact on overall quality of care.

One easy to understand measure is nurse-to-patient ratios. The evidence shows that higher nurse staffing—independent of environment or disease—improves patient outcomes. For instance, one study showed that in a hospital at capacity, a 10% increase in the number of patients assigned to a nurse leads to a 28% increase in adverse events such as infections and medication errors[39] (i.e., fewer nurses with higher patient loads lead to more adverse events); on the other hand, in another study, a 10% increase in RNs was associated with a 9.5% decrease in the odds of patients developing pneumonia[40] (i.e., more nurses lead to decreased adverse events).

Thus, improving nurse employment, job satisfaction, skill level, and work processes are all focuses of quality initiatives and policy-making. In particular, you can look to the National Quality Forum and The Joint Commission for policy prescriptions.

Everyone interested in a more extensive introduction to safety in health care should read the AHRQ's Patient Safety Primers at *[psnet. ahrq.gov/primerHome.aspx]*.

Health Information Technology

Defining Terms

Health care communication and data-sharing systems at most institutions are stuck in the pagers-and-faxes era (unfortunately, they've ditched the acid-washed jeans). However, health information technology (health IT) is a booming field making big changes, due largely to new incentives (see "Meaningful Use" below) and to creative IT professionals working to drag the health care system into the 21st century.

Health IT is a simple concept: the application of electronic systems to organizing and using health data, from charting to writing prescriptions to transmitting MRI results digitally. However, as with many aspects of health care, this simple concept quickly becomes extremely complicated when put into practice. At its most basic level, health IT refers to electronic health records (EHRs or EMRs), systems for charting, coding, and prescribing electronically—but it also encompasses the exchange of health information across systems, telemedicine, and even tools that will help providers avoid mistakes and make the best diagnostic decisions.

In general, you can think of health IT as the use of technology not just to make health care more efficient and less error-prone, but rather—on a grander scale—to transform the way that we use health information to make delivery of care better and more effective. However, as we discuss at the end of this section, health IT must be viewed as just one part of trans-forming health care delivery.

Electronic Health Records in Context

In 2012, surveys showed that 44% of general hospitals had at least a basic EHR, and 17% had a comprehensive system.[41] (This is pretty incredible if you consider that, in 2008, before the HITECH Act, only 10% of hospitals had a basic EHR.[42] Score one for incentives.) More of these systems are more likely

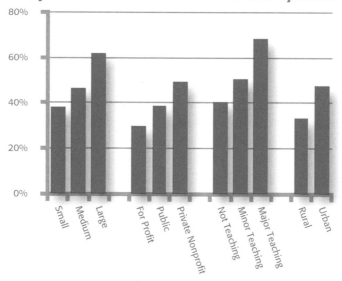

Adoption of Electronic Health Record Systems

Adapted from: DesRoches, et al., "Adoption of Electronic Health Records Grows Rapidly, But Fewer Than Half of US Hospitals Had at Least a Basic System In 2012," August 2013. Note: Data from 2012.

to be large, urban, teaching hospitals, while rural and for-profit hospitals lag behind.[41] Further, the use of EHR is growing within outpatient medical practices, particularly if they are larger or integrated with a hospital system.[43]

A major challenge is that more than 500 companies make EHR software,[44] producing a lot of competition. Thus, hospitals and practices have a lot of options, but they also are likely to be using incompatible systems that cannot easily share data with each other.

The ability to share data is called interoperability, defined more specifically as "the ability of different information technology systems and software applications to communicate, exchange data, and use the information that has been exchanged."[45] It is also a major goal of health IT, as a step toward better health outcomes. Interoperability is very important in allowing different systems to work together, increasing efficiency, improving patient transfers, decreasing repeated tests, and, long-term, to creating standards for clinical decision-making nationwide. (See the Health Information Exchange section below for more information.) A good example of interoperability is the Blue Button initiative at the Veterans Administration, which allows patients to download their charts for use, as well as for non-VA facilities to receive health summaries.[46]

There are many options for EHRs, but a few vendors dominate the market. The leaders in the inpatient and outpatient settings are:[47]

Outpatient	Inpatient
▸ Epic Systems, 20% market share	▸ Epic Systems, 19% market share
▸ Allscripts, 11%	▸ MEDITECH, 17%
▸ eClinicalWorks LLC, 8%	▸ Computer Programs and Systems, 14%
▸ NextGen Healthcare, 7%	▸ Cerner Corporation, 9%
▸ GE Healthcare, 6%	▸ McKesson, 9%

Computerized Physician Order Entry

Computerized Physician Order Entry (CPOE) is software built on top of basic EHR features that allows providers to prescribe medications, order tests, and give other types of instructions electronically. The goal of CPOE is to improve safety and efficiency. The benefits of electronic orders are multiple and obvious—aside from releasing everyone from the tyranny of bad doctor handwriting. CPOE shortens work process delays, makes instructions easier to access, groups multiple common orders in sets, and can catch mistakes (i.e., a clear overdose, or a bad drug interaction). Seventy-two percent of hospitals used CPOE in 2012, a huge leap from 2008, when it was only 27%—again, due in part to the HITECH incentives.[48]

Often, when a provider wants to make an order, he or she doesn't just want one thing but wants several things that tend to go together. Thus the "order set,"[49] a controversial aspect of CPOE systems. An order set is a pre-defined list of orders that are most common (or suggested as a best practice) for a particular diagnosis or situation. On the plus side, an order set is efficient, evidence-based, and doesn't rely on faulty memories. On the down side, the order set doesn't always account for unique circumstances or preferences, which is frustrating to a busy provider who doesn't know how to bypass the system. This is an area in which greater input from users should improve accessibility and make order sets a significant contributor over time.

Clinical Decision Support

Clinical decision support (CDS) refers to technology which uses data to help providers make decisions regarding patient care. It is, however, not only a vague term but a vague concept. CDS can help with decisions about medication prescribing, adherence to guidelines, and making diagnoses. Examples of CDS tools in an EHR for prescribing medications include checking a medication against patient data such as allergies, renal function, and other medications. An EHR can display appropriate dosing to a prescriber or pop up warnings about allergies and dangerous interactions. One step up would be a CDS that alerts providers to patients who, because they have certain conditions, would benefit from a particular intervention, like notifying a provider which of their heart failure patients would benefit from a pacemaker. Another step up would be a diagnostic tool such as DiagnosisPro, a website which will provide a differential diagnosis for lists of symptoms. (You can check this out at <http://en.diagnosispro.com/>). Such advanced CDS tools are exciting for the future but not exactly sophisticated at this point.

Meaningful Use

The HITECH Act in 2009 set up a program through the Centers for Medicare & Medicaid Services (CMS) to incentivize the growth of EHR through monetary rewards—and, later, penalties—tied to a set of standards or objectives termed "meaningful use."[50] The program began in 2011, and the last year to enroll is 2014. Individual providers (such as physicians or dentists) and institutions (such as hospitals) can enroll. By 2012, more than 3,000 hospitals had enrolled in the incentive program, and 800 had received a total of $1.4 billion in payments.[51]

The incentive program is to be rolled out in three stages. These stages are outlined in the graphic below.[52]

Stage 1: 2011-2012 Data capture and sharing	Stage 2: 2014 Advance clinical processes	Stage 3: 2016 Improved outcomes
Meaningful use criteria focus on:		
▸ Electronically capturing health information in a standardized format	▸ More rigorous health information exchange (HIE)	▸ Improving quality, safety, and efficiency, leading to improved health outcomes
▸ Using that information to track key clinical conditions	▸ Increased requirements for e-prescribing and incorporating lab results	▸ Decision support for national high-priority conditions
▸ Communicating that information for care coordination processes	▸ Electronic transmission of patient care summaries across multiple settings	▸ Patient access to self-management tools
▸ Initiating the reporting of clinical quality measures and public health information	▸ More patient-controlled data	▸ Access to comprehensive patient data through patient-centered HIE
▸ Using information to engage patients and their families in their care		▸ Improving population health

Further, CMS has released four regulations defining "meaningful use." There are 14 "core objectives" for Stage 1. In 2012, only 42% of hospitals could meet all 14 Stage 1 criteria (and those that did were more likely to be large, urban, teaching, private, nonprofits), whereas only 5% could meet all of the Stage 2 criteria.[41] Keep in mind also that the stakes are higher for hospitals and providers than just missing out on bonus incentive payments: There are penalties, too, which will start in 2015.[53]

Health Information Exchange

All of the above sections describe tools or concepts that work within a single organization. To share data between hospitals or medical practices, we have Health Information Exchange (HIE). Put very simply, HIE is about sharing data between EHRs. If providers can see information about a patient from outside your own organization, in a standardized format, they are in a better position to make diagnosis and treatment decisions. Further, data sharing can set industry standards—if you can see what other provider practices and outcomes are, then you are in a better position to improve your own practices and outcomes. This applies to measures in health care safety, quality, cost, and clinical standards. But data sharing is not easy: Barriers to HIE include the cultural (health care systems that do not wish to share data, for various reasons), technological (as we discussed earlier in the section, many EHRs lack interoperability and are therefore "blind" to each other), privacy (how do you make the data relevant without violating patient privacy), and financial (overcoming those other barriers costs money).

One example of HIE was established in 2004, the Nationwide Health Information Network (NwHIN or NHIN). The NHIN is a "network of networks," with 24 participants. In February 2009, the Social Security Administration and MedVirginia became the first organizations to share data, and since then the Department of Veterans Affairs, the Department of Defense, and Kaiser Permanente began sharing data, as well.[54] Eventually, many more entities should be able to access data for research, standard-setting, and quality improvement initiatives. However, HIE is still taking baby steps, and its promise lies largely in the future.[55]

Health IT and Outcomes

So far, all of this sounds pretty good. Who could argue with CPOE, which eliminates handwriting errors, and CDS, which catches dangerous drug interactions? What physician is unhappy about checking a computer for a test result rather than running across the hospital looking at charts all day? What patient is upset that his or her information is available 24/7 in a portal?

It makes sense and seems obvious, but, in health care, you get yourself into trouble if you trust things that make sense without checking to see if they really work. Switching to an EHR from a paper charting system takes a lot of money (we mean a LOT of money), in addition to time training and lost efficiency as providers learn the new system, so the outcomes better be worth the investment. What does the evidence say? Do EHRs really improve outcomes?

The evidence has been conflicting and controversial, but in any case it's not a slam-dunk for health IT. For instance, in 2010, a large study showed "no significant relationship" between EHR use and improved quality of care for heart attacks, congestive heart failure, or pneumonia, though there was some improvement in prevention of surgical complications.[41] Likewise, the study didn't show any decrease in length-of-stay, 30-day readmission rates, or inpatient costs.[41] In 2013, another study showed modest improvements in 30-day mortality, inpatient mortality, length-of-stay, with a worsening of readmission rates.[56]

Why aren't we always seeing the expected improvements? Many reasons have been suggested. Possibly because we haven't given health care staff enough time to acclimate to the new way of working. Perhaps because the technology hasn't been made to best fit the way providers work. Perhaps because not enough providers use these new systems yet. Perhaps because EHR really isn't enough—we need the data-sharing promise of HIE to truly change the way work processes affect quality of care. Perhaps because technology is simply a tool to change behavior. (See "Culture Change" below.)

What's clear is that health IT has become a major force in health care, and that isn't going to change. Equally clear, though, is that health IT is not a deux ex machina that will save health care. There are more barriers to overcome and more evidence to be gathered.

Culture Change

Quality and technology innovations have the potential to revolutionize the delivery of care and greatly improve patient outcomes. Two prominent innovations we have mentioned are checklists and Electronic Health Records (EHRs); both have great promise but neither has yet demonstrated a conclusive improvement in patient outcomes. That is perhaps because a checklist or an EHR is just one tool within a larger organizational culture that needs to change.

An analogy would be a person who wants to get fit and healthy and buys a thighmaster. Fifteen minutes a day, he uses the thighmaster, but the rest of the day he continues to eat junk food and sit on the couch. We all know that's not going to work (much to the authors' chagrin). Although the thighmaster "works" as expected, without a change in his other behaviors and actions he will not obtain the outcome desired. The same issue applies with quality and technology innovations. As Lucien Leape says about checklists, "the key is recognizing that changing practice is not a technical problem that can be solved by ticking off boxes on a checklist but a social problem of human behavior and interaction."[57]

Susan DeVore and Keith Figoli wrote that "Health IT implementation represents a sweeping change away from business as usual to an entirely new approach in health care—one that will require process and behavior changes from nearly all health care workers. As such, it's important to see the effort as an exercise in change management, not an IT initiative."[58] This is the real challenge of health quality and technology innovations. Keep this in mind when you read about new software tools that are going to totally fix health care—and when you read a few months later that they don't live up to expectations.

Patient Privacy and the Law

If you work in the health professions, you will most certainly have to learn more about the Health Insurance Portability and Accountability Act (HIPAA), which in 2003 became the first universal code in the U.S. to protect patient privacy. HIPAA protects patient confidentiality and informed consent, regulating how patients' personal health information can be viewed, stored, and used in both clinical care and in research.

The focus is on health information (i.e., any information about a patient's health) that can be identified as referring to a particular patient. This is called "Protected Health Information."[59] Thus, health information can be used—for instance, for research or quality improvement initiatives—but only if the information is "deidentified," that is, someone couldn't figure out who the information referred to. Identifiers include name, social security number, geographic location (anything more specific than state), any date associated with the patient or patient's stay, medical record number, telephone number, email address, or insurance number (the list goes on).

All health care workers must undergo regular HIPAA education and training, and hospitals must maintain an entire administrative infrastructure dedicated to HIPAA requirements. Violating HIPAA is a criminal offense, with tiered penalties. However, very few penalties are actually given, as seen in the figure below.[60,61]

96,000 cases reported

22,000 cases required action

526 CASES HANDLED BY THE DEPARTMENT OF JUSTICE

13 FINES GIVEN BY THE DEPARTMENT OF JUSTICE

As you might imagine, HIPAA is not without critics. Some of the arguments against the law—not against patient privacy protection, but rather against the specifics of HIPAA—are as follows:

▸ The multitude of regulations is too confusing, so institutions err on the side of never giving out any information, even when it's allowed by the law.

- HIPAA requires too much administrative overhead in order for institutions to be compliant.
- It hinders biomedical and population-based research, by making it too costly and time-consuming.[62]
- It may limit the communication necessary for good care, particularly for those with caregivers (like the elderly) or who may need more social support (like the mentally ill).[63]
- It hinders the burgeoning field of health IT, from electronic health records to mobile apps.[64,65]
- It's unrealistic for the workflow of a hospital and gets violated constantly, reducing efficiency without significantly increasing patient privacy.

Protecting patient privacy is extremely important. It is also an increasing concern, as electronic health records, mobile apps, and health information exchange create networks in which ever larger breaches of patient data are possible. For better or for worse, it's not just HIPAA that limits innovation in health IT—it's patient privacy.

Medical Malpractice *with Brian Yagi*

Patients who believe they have been injured in some way by a health care provider can file a medical malpractice claim. To prove malpractice, the patient must show that the injury was caused by the provider's negligence, meaning that he or she didn't practice medicine consistent with the accepted medico–legal standard of care. If a patient wins a case or a favorable settlement, the health care provider, through insurance, may have to compensate the patient for loss of income due to injury and for noneconomic losses, such as pain and suffering. Although most malpractice claims are made against physicians, claims can be brought against any health care provider, including students. To protect against the financial risk of future malpractice lawsuits, most physicians purchase malpractice insurance. Hospitals and health care networks often purchase insurance for their employees, while independent physicians typically purchase their own policies.

Medical malpractice serves two goals: (1) to compensate victims of poor medical care, and (2) to encourage safe and responsible medical practice. Our current system is designed to accomplish both by punishing negligent providers through the court system (called "torts"). Some question whether it wouldn't be better to handle each goal separately, and to focus on the system rather than on individuals.

A few key facts about medical malpractice:

▸ More than 75% of physicians will have at least one malpractice claim brought against them by the age of 65. For those in high-risk specialties such as general surgery, the rate is 99%.[66]

▸ The cost of malpractice insurance varies dramatically by location and specialty. Premiums for a general internist in Minnesota run around $3,500 per year, while those for OB/GYNs in Long Island, NY cost $225,000 or more.[67]

▸ The overwhelming majority of patients who receive negligent care don't file malpractice claims.[68]

▸ Only one-fifth of malpractice claims result in payment to the patient; the average payment is $275,000. However, proving that there's no liability isn't cheap either—averaging $110,000 for a successful trial defense, and $27,000 even if the claim is dropped, withdrawn, or dismissed before making it to the courtroom.[69]

▸ Americans file more malpractice claims than patients in other countries—four times as many as Canadians, for example.[70]

Problems

COSTS TO PROVIDERS

These costs are both economic and psychological. Some physicians pay exorbitant rates for their malpractice insurance. Economically, this may inhibit a physician's ability to maintain a private practice and affect what field she or he chooses to enter. Many physicians think malpractice insurance premiums are a major problem.

COSTS TO SYSTEM

The fear of litigation has caused a shift in the way that physicians provide care to patients, which is known as "defensive medicine." There are two types of defensive medicine: positive, in which physicians overuse services to "cover their bases" in case of a lawsuit, rather than to practice good medicine; and negative, in which physicians avoid high-risk patients and procedures they fear could be a higher risk for litigation. This isn't just a theoretical problem—in recent surveys, more than four out of five specialist physicians report practicing positive defensive medicine.[71,72] This can have deleterious effects:

▸ **Questionable quality:** Positive defensive medicine leads to the use of tests and procedures, such as MRIs or colonoscopies, when not medically necessary. Not only can this expose patients to procedural risks for very little possibility of a finding, but it also may turn up benign findings, leading to more procedures and more risks— providing no increased, and perhaps even decreased, health benefit.

▸ **Increased cost:** Defensive medicine is how medical malpractice indirectly raises health care costs, as the above-mentioned tests and procedures tend to be very expensive. Although calculating the true cost of the medical liability system is an inexact science, a recent study by researchers at Harvard estimated that the total cost in 2008 was $55 billion—$47 billion of which is due to defensive medicine— in hospital services and physician and clinical (outpatient) services, accounting for 2.4% of total health care spending.[73]

COSTS TO PATIENTS

Patients without good insurance coverage will often end up paying very large bills, in part due to defensive medicine (for instance, the average cost of an ED visit in 2011 was $1,354).[74] In addition, if patients do encounter medical errors, it's extremely unlikely that they will receive a malpractice pay-out. Several barriers are in their way:

▸ A patient has to convince a lawyer to take on his or her case. Considering that most malpractice plaintiffs' lawyers are paid via a percentage of the settlement, and considering the high costs of litigating malpractice lawsuits regardless of the victor, patients must have clear-cut cases with large damages to entice most lawyers. This means that most patients who experience medical errors face difficulties in establishing lawsuits and thus have no recourse for compensation.

▸ Patients must convince juries to find in their favor. Regardless of the reasons, right or wrong, this just isn't likely: Most claims are settled, withdrawn, or dropped before making it to trial, and most of those that do go to a jury trial are found in favor of the physician. According to a recent study, "physicians win 80% to 90% of the jury trials with weak evidence of medical negligence, approximately 70% of the borderline cases, and even 50% of the trials in cases with strong evidence of medical negligence."[75]

In addition, many feel that the psychological environment created by our current system of medical malpractice erodes the trusting relationship necessary for good medicine—which is bad for both providers and patients.

Potential Reforms

ARBITRATION

Arbitration is the determination of a dispute *not* through the court system but rather by an impartial referee (the arbitrator) agreed upon by both parties. A growing trend among clinics and hospitals is to make arbitration agreements mandatory, meaning that patients must use an arbitrator and can't later sue for damages.

The benefits of this system are that costs are kept low for both parties, arbitrations can happen more quickly than lawsuits, and patients don't need "rainmaker" cases to convince lawyers to represent them. The drawbacks of this system are that some institutions pressure patients to sign binding arbitration agreements before receiving care, arbitration pay-outs are often capped at levels that may be low (i.e., $250,000), and providers may reject arbitrators who decide in favor of patients too often.

DISCLOSURE AND OFFER

Several private insurers and university health care systems have decided to avoid the judicial system by handling medical injuries internally. When a patient suffers an unexpected injury, the institution launches an internal investigation to determine whether it was the result of medical error. If it turns out the injury was the result of error or malpractice, the institution discloses that fact to the patient with as much transparency as possible. It then offers a settlement to that patient, roughly commensurate with (but usually below) the expected outcome of a trial.[76] The patient must sign away his or her right to sue if accepting the settlement offer. This system marks a philosophical shift for physicians towards a "disclose and offer" system as opposed to "deny and defend." The University of Michigan has implemented such a system and seen dramatic decreases in the number of claims filed by patients.[77] Most important, it has learned from its investigations and implemented several institutional reforms that have led to increased patient safety.

HEALTH COURTS

Philip Howard, a New York attorney and founder of the legal reform organization Common Good, suggests keeping the courts but bypassing the juries. In Howard's conception, "Expert judges with special training would resolve health care disputes. They would issue written rulings providing guidance on proper standards of care. These rulings would set precedents on which both patients and physicians could rely. As with existing administrative courts in other areas of law—for tax disputes, workers' compensation, and vaccine liability, among others—there would be no juries. Each ruling could be appealed to a new medical appeals court."[78] Indeed, New Zealand, Sweden, and Denmark all have health courts that have proven effective at implementing a diverse array of patient safety mechanisms.[79]

TORT REFORM

In general, tort reform seeks to cap damage pay-outs and block frivolous lawsuits. California was the first to enact tort reform, in 1975, when it passed the Medical Injury Compensation Reform Act. This act contains five stipulations:
- Noneconomic damages are capped at $250,000
- Attorneys' fees are capped
- The statute of limitations on medical errors is shortened
- Arbitration is binding
- Physicians can pay damages in installments rather than in a lump sum

Many other states have enacted tort reform in varying ways, including 30 that limit noneconomic damages.[80] Proponents of these reforms claim that they reduce the number of frivolous lawsuits as well as the emphasis on defensive medicine. Opponents claim that, in addition to punishing patients whose damages truly are higher than the cap, they're ineffective in reducing medical errors and costs.

SUMMARY

Medical malpractice and how to fix it appears to be a mess—a crucially important mess, based on how often it comes up in society. Which raises the question: Is the problem overstated?

Health services researcher Aaron Carroll made the graph shown below to illustrate the costs of medical malpractice in the context of total health spending.[81] While the costs of defensive medicine—$47 billion—are nothing to sneeze at, it's also clearly not the primary driver of high health costs. Accordingly, Carroll indicates that tort reform will do little to reduce costs.

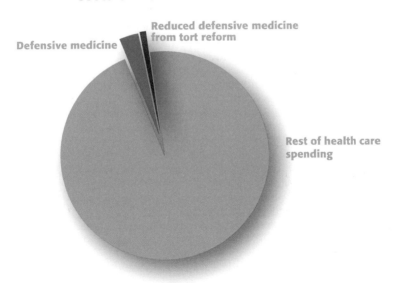

Costs of Defensive Medicine

Defensive medicine

Reduced defensive medicine from tort reform

Rest of health care spending

Aaron Carroll, "Meme-busting: Tort reform = cost control," June 2011.
Used with permission.

References

1. Davis MM, Taubert K, et al. Influenza Vaccination as Secondary Prevention for Cardiovascular Disease. *Circulation.* 2006;114(14):1549.
2. MacIntyre CR, Heywood AE, et al. Ischaemic heart disease, influenza and influenza vaccination: a prospective case–control study. *Heart.* 2013;99(24):1843-8
3. Gonzales R, Steiner JF, et al. Antibiotic Prescribing for Adults with Colds, Upper Respiratory Tract Infections, and Bronchitis by Ambulatory Care Physicians. *JAMA: The Journal of the American Medical Association.* 1997;278(11):901.
4. Landrigan CP, Parry GJ, et al. Temporal Trends in Rates of Patient Harm Resulting from Medical Care. *New England Journal of Medicine.* 2010;363(22):2124.
5. Friedly J, Chan L, et al. Geographic Variation in Epidural Steroid Injection Use in Medicare Patients. *The Journal of Bone and Joint Surgery.* 2008;90(8):1730.
6. Agency for Healthcare Research and Quality. Module 6: The Way Forward—Promoting Quality Improvement in the States. www.ahrq.gov/professionals/quality-patient-safety/quality-resources/tools/diabguide/diabqguidemod6.html. Accessed June 18, 2014.
7. Mitchell P. Defining Patient Safety and Quality Care. The Agency for Healthcare Research and Quality.
8. Classen DC, Resar R, et al. 'Global Trigger Tool' Shows That Adverse Events in Hospitals May Be Ten Times Greater Than Previously Measured. *Health Affairs.* Apr 2011;30(4):581.
9. Kohn LT, Corrigan J, et al. *To Err Is Human: Building a Safer Health System.* Vol 6: Natl Academy Pr; 2000.
10. National Center for Injury Prevention and Control. Wisqars Leading Causes of Death Reports. webappa.cdc.gov/sasweb/ncipc/leadcaus10.html. Accessed June 28, 2014.
11. AHRQ. The National Quality Strategy. www.ahrq.gov/workingforquality/. Accessed June 28, 2014.
12. The Joint Commission. National Patient Safety Goals. www.jointcommission.org/standards_information/npsgs.aspx. Accessed June 28, 2014.
13. National Quality Forum. Safe Practices for Better Healthcare. www.qualityforum.org/Publications/2010/04/Safe_Practices_for_Better_Healthcare_%E2%80%93_2010_Update.aspx. Accessed June 28, 2014.
14. Agency for Healthcare Research and Quality. AHRQ Patient Safety Network—Medication Errors. psnet.ahrq.gov/primer.aspx?primerID=23. Accessed June 23, 2014.
15. Bonsall L. 8 Rights of Medication Administration. www.nursingcenter.com/Blog/post/2011/05/27/8-rights-of-medication-administration.aspx. Accessed June 23, 2014.
16. Van Den Bos J, Rustagi K, et al. The $17.1 billion Problem: The Annual Cost of Measurable Medical Errors. *Health Affairs.* 2011-04-01 2011;30(4):596.
17. Binder L. Do as Dr. House Doesn't. stream.wsj.com/story/experts-journal-reports/SS-2-135503/SS-2-207380/. Accessed June 23, 2014.
18. Vidyarthi AR, Arora V, et al. Managing Discontinuity in Academic Medical Centers: Strategies for a Safe and Effective Resident Sign-Out. *Journal of Hospital Medicine.* 2006;1(4):257.
19. Starmer A, Spector N, et al. I-Pass, a Mnemonic to Standardize Verbal Handoffs. *American Academy of Pediatrics.* 2012-02-01 2012;129(2):201.
20. Cohen MD, Hilligoss PB. The Published Literature on Handoffs in Hospitals: Deficiencies Identified in an Extensive Review. *Quality & Safety in Health Care.* Dec 2010;19(6):493.
21. Horwitz LI. Does Improving Handoffs Reduce Medical Error Rates? *JAMA: The Journal of the American Medical Association.* 2013;310(21):2255.

22. Agency for Healthcare Research and Quality. AHRQ Patient Safety Network—Adverse Events after Hospital Discharge. psnet.ahrq.gov/primer.aspx?primerID=11. Accessed June 20, 2014.

23. Centers for Medicare & Medicaid Services. National Medicare Readmission Findings: Recent Data and Trends. www.academyhealth.org/files/2012/sunday/brennan.pdf. Accessed June 23, 2014.

24. Agency for Healthcare Research and Quality. Medication Reconciliation. psnet.ahrq.gov/primer.aspx?primerID=1. Accessed June 19, 2014.

25. Volpp KG, Rosen AK, et al. Mortality Among Hospitalized Medicare Beneficiaries in the First 2 Years Following ACGME Resident Duty Hour Reform. *JAMA: The Journal of the American Medical Association.* 2007;298(9):975-983.

26. Institute of Medicine. *Resident Duty Hours: Enhancing Sleep, Supervision, and Safety.* Washington, DC. 2008.

27. Singh H, Thomas EJ, et al. Medical Errors Involving Trainees: A Study of Closed Malpractice Claims from 5 Insurers. *Archives of Internal Medicine.* 2007;167(19):2030.

28. Volpp KG, Rosen AK, et al. Mortality among Hospitalized Medicare Beneficiaries in the First 2 Years Following ACGME Resident Duty Hour Reform. *JAMA: The Journal of the American Medical Association.* 2007;298(9):975.

29. Pronovost P ND, Berenholtz S, et al. An Intervention to Decrease Catheter-Related Bloodstream Infections in the ICU. *New England Journal of Medicine.* 2006;355:2725.

30. Urbach D, Govindarajan, Anand, Saskin, Refik, et al. Introduction of Surgical Safety Checklists in Ontario, Canada. *New England Journal of Medicine.* 2014;370:1029.

31. Forum NQ. List of SREs. www.qualityforum.org/topics/sres/list_of_sres.aspx. Accessed June 28, 2014.

32. Lembitz A, Clarke TJ. Clarifying "Never Events" and Introducing "Always Events." *Patient Saf Surg.* 2009;3:26.

33. Division of Health Care Quality. Serious Reportable Event (SREs). www.mass.gov/eohhs/gov/departments/dph/programs/hcq/serious-reportable-event-sres.html. Accessed June 28, 2014.

34. Centers for Disease Control and Prevention. Data and Statistics. www.cdc.gov/hai/surveillance/. Accessed June 19, 2014.

35. Scott RD. The Direct Medical Costs of Healthcare-Associated Infections in US Hospitals and the Benefits of Prevention. www.cdc.gov/hai/pdfs/hai/scott_costpaper.pdf. Accessed June 28, 2014.

36. Department of Health and Human Services. Hospital-Acquired Conditions (HAC) in Acute Inpatient Prospective Payment System (IPPS) Hospitals. www.cms.gov/Medicare/Medicare-Fee-for-Service-Payment/HospitalAcqCond/downloads/HACFactSheet.pdf. Accessed June 23, 2014.

37. Allegranzi B, Pittet D. Role of Hand Hygiene in Healthcare-Associated Infection Prevention. *Journal of Hospital Infection.* 2009;73(4):305.

38. Erasmus V, Daha T, et al. Systematic Review of Studies on Compliance with Hand Hygiene Guidelines in Hospital Care. *Infection Control and Hospital Epidemiology.* 2010;31(3):283.

39. Weissman J, Rothschild J, et al. Hospital Workload and Adverse Events. *Medical Care.* 2014;45(5):448.

40. Cho SH, Ketefian S, et al. The Effects of Nurse Staffing on Adverse Events, Morbidity, Mortality, and Medical Costs. *Nursing research.* Mar-Apr 2003;52(2):71.

41. DesRoches C, Charles D, et al. Adoption of Electronic Health Records Grows Rapidly, but Fewer Than Half of US Hospitals Had at Least a Basic System in 2012. *Health Affairs.* 2013-08-01 2013;32(8):1478.

42. Jha AK, DesRoches CM, et al. Use of Electronic Health Records in US Hospitals. *New England Journal of Medicine.* 2009;360(16):1628.

43. Audet AM SD, Doty MM. Where Are We on the Diffusion Curve? Trends and Drives of Primary Care Physicians' Use of Health Information Technology. *Health Services Research.* 2014;49(1pt2):347.

44. Verdon D. Top 100 EHRs: Why Understanding a Company's Financial Performance Today May Influence Purchasing Decisions Tomorrow. *Medical Economics.* 2013-10-25 2013.

45. Healthcare Information and Management Systems Society. What Is Interoperability? www.himss.org/library/interoperability-standards/what-is? Accessed June 23, 2014.

46. U.S. Department of Veterans Affairs. Blue Button Home. www4.va.gov/bluebutton/. Accessed June 13, 2014.

47. Software Advice. EHR Meaningful Use Market Share Industryview. www.softwareadvice.com/medical/industryview/ehr-meaningful-use-market-share-2014/. Accessed June 23, 2014.

48. The Office of the National Coordinator for Health Information Technology. *Onc Data Brief.* www.healthit.gov/sites/default/files/oncdatabrief10final.pdf. Accessed June 23, 2014.

49. Bobb AM, Payne TH, et al. Viewpoint: Controversies Surrounding Use of Order Sets for Clinical Decision Support in Computerized Provider Order Entry. *J Am Med Inform Assoc.* Jan-Feb 2007;14(1):41.

50. Blumenthal D. The "Meaningful Use" Regulation for Electronic Health Records. *New England Journal of Medicine.* 2010;363:501.

51. DesRoches CM, Worzala C, et al. Small, Nonteaching, and Rural Hospitals Continue to Be Slow in Adopting Electronic Health Record Systems. *Health Affairs.* May 2012;31(5):1092.

52. HealthIT.gov. How to Attain Meaningful Use. www.healthit.gov/providers-professionals/how-attain-meaningful-use. Accessed June 23, 2014.

53. HealthIT.gov. Are There Penalties for Providers Who Don't Switch to Electronic Health Records (EHR)? www.healthit.gov/providers-professionals/faqs/are-there-penalties-providers-who-don%E2%80%99t-switch-electronic-health-record. Accessed June 23, 2014.

54. Nationwide Health Information Network. What Is the NHIN? www.healthit.gov/sites/default/files/what-Is-the-nhin--2.pdf. Accessed June 19, 2014.

55. McDonald CJ, Overhage JM, et al. The Indiana Network for Patient Care: A Working Local Health Information Infrastructure. *Health Affairs.* 2005-09-01 2005;24(5):1214.

56. Lee J, Kuo Y-F, et al. The Effect of Electronic Medical Record Adoption on Outcomes in US Hospitals. *BMC Health Services Research.* 2013;13(1):39.

57. Leape L. The Checklist Conundrum. *New England Journal of Medicine.* 2014;370:1063.

58. DeVore S, Figlioli K. Lessons Premier Hospitals Learned About Implementing Electronic Health Records. *Health Affairs.* 2010-04-01 2010;29(4):664.

59. U.S. Department of Health & Human Services. Summary of the HIPAA Privacy Rule. www.hhs.gov/ocr/privacy/hipaa/understanding/summary/. Accessed June 19, 2014.

60. Chesanow N. Is HIPAA Creating More Problems Than It's Preventing?: What Can You Reveal, What Do You Risk? www.medscape.com/viewarticle/810648_2. Accessed June 28, 2014.

61. Melamedia LLC. Health Information Privacy/Security Alert. melamedia.com/shopsite_sc/store/html/hipa_intro.html. Accessed June 19, 2014.

62. Ness RB. Influence of the HIPAA Privacy Rule on Health Research. *JAMA: The Journal of the American Medical Association.* Nov. 14, 2007;298(18):2164.

63. Marbury D. HIPAA Hinders Patients' Wish to Share Online Health Records with Care Partners, Report Says. *Medical Economics eConsult.* medicaleconomics.modernmedicine.com/medical-economics/news/hipaa-hinders-patients-wish-share-online-health-records-care-partners-report-.

64. Gregg H. HIPAA Hinders Big Data Innovation. www.beckershospitalreview.com/healthcare-information-technology/report-hipaa-hinders-big-data-innovation.html. Accessed June 19, 2014.

65. McCann E. HIPAA Breaches in Top 5 Security Worries. www.healthcareitnews.com/news/hipaa-breaches-among-top-5-security-concerns-new-year. Accessed June 19, 2014.

66. Jena AB, Seabury S, et al. Malpractice Risk According to Physician Specialty. *New England Journal of Medicine.* 2011;365(7):629.

67. Lowes R. Malpractice Premiums Drop for 6th Straight Year. 2014. www.medscape.com/viewarticle/812451.

68. Studdert DM, Thomas EJ, et al. Negligent Care and Malpractice Claiming Behavior in Utah and Colorado. *Medical care.* 2000;38(3):250.

69. Carroll A, Parikh P, et al. The Impact of Defense Expenses in Medical Malpractice Claims,. *J Law Med Ethics.* 2012;40(1):135.

70. Anderson GF, Hussey PS, et al. Health Spending in the United States and the Rest of the Industrialized World. *Health Affairs.* 2005;24(4):903.

71. Massachusetts Medical Society. Investigation of Defensive Medicine in Massachusetts. www.ncrponline.org/PDFs/2008/Mass_Med_Soc.pdf. Accessed June 28, 2014.

72. Studdert DM, Mello MM, et al. Defensive Medicine among High-Risk Specialist Physicians in a Volatile Malpractice Environment. *JAMA: The Journal of the American Medical Association.* 2005;293(21):2609.

73. Mello MM, Chandra A, et al. National Costs of the Medical Liability System. *Health Affairs.* 2010;29(9):1569.

74. Agency for Healthcare Research and Quality. Medical Expenditure Panel Survey. meps. ahrq.gov/mepsweb/index.jsp. Accessed June 19, 2014.

75. Peters P. The Case for Medical Liability Reform. *Symposium: Clinical Risk and Judicial Reasoning.* 2008;467(2):352.

76. Mello M, Gallagher T. Malpractice Reform—Opportunities for Leadership by Health Care Institutions and Liability Insurers. *New England Journal of Medicine.* 2010;362:1353.

77. Boothman R, Blackwell A, et al. A Better Aproach to Medical Malpractice Claims? The University of Michigan Experience. *Journal of Health and Life Sciences Law.* 2009;2(2):1.

78. Common Good. Establish Health Courts. www.commongood.org/pages/establish-health-courts. Accessed June 28, 2014.

79. Mello MM, Studdert DM, et al. "Health Courts" and Accountability for Patient Safety. *Milbank Quarterly.* 2006;84(3):459.

80. American Tort Reform Association. Noneconomic Damages Reform. www.atra.org/issues/noneconomic-damages-reform. Accessed June 19, 2014.

81. Carroll A. Meme-Busting: Tort Reform = Cost Control. theincidentaleconomist.com/wordpress/meme-busting-tort-reform-cost-control-2/. Accessed June 28, 2014.

Chapter 4
Research, Pharmaceuticals, and Medical Devices

Many books about health care and health policy skip over information on research, pharmaceuticals, and medical devices. However, these industries form the backbone of health care. In this chapter, you'll gain an overview of these important topics. Keep in mind, though, that this entire book is designed to be an overview rather than an in-depth study—many, many books have been filled with information we omit, which is especially true for this chapter.

> **Authors' note:** This chapter focuses on problems and issues in the world of research, pharmaceuticals, and devices but doesn't devote the same space to the incredible advancements in knowledge and practice in these areas. We highlight problems in this book's limited space because they're less likely to be familiar to the average reader. For a more complete picture of the positives and negatives of these industries, please see the Suggested Reading section on page 224.

Research

Types of Research

BASIC RESEARCH

You can think of basic scientific research as the pure quest for knowledge, which covers an enormous range—from cellular components to organ structure and function, and from the interactions among organ systems to behavioral science. Being pre-clinical, basic research usually takes place in a lab and involves living cells, tissue, viruses, bacteria, and animals. Some examples of basic research include stem cell research, visualizing the structure of a viral envelope, sequencing a section of DNA, and finding the cellular mutations that cause cancer.

Some basic research may end up without any practical application; some—like the discovery of penicillin's bactericidal effects—may revolutionize medicine. The famous biologist Richard Dawkins wrote that basic science research "might be no use for anything at present, but it has great potential for the future."[1]

APPLIED RESEARCH

Applied research is similar to basic research, but with a practical goal in mind. You can think of applied research as science with a direct purpose or application, or a quest to solve problems we already know about. Examples include developing gene therapies, testing potential cancer drugs, and developing vaccines.

One type of applied research, known as translational research, focuses specifically on applying basic science to human illness. Translational research usually includes multidisciplinary teams who work on different aspects of guiding the research process "from bench to bedside." Recent years have seen a big push for translational research; in 2011 the National Center for Advancing Translational Sciences became the newest center of the National Institutes of Health (NIH).

Basic and applied research necessarily overlap and feed into each other. For instance, the Human Genome Project involved a lot of research that is rapidly being applied in terms of diagnosis and disease processes, but many of the project's applications remain to be discovered. Though immediate aims may not be obvious for all of genetics research, the impetus for sequencing the human genome is that it will be useful someday for developing new therapies to treat human disease.

CLINICAL RESEARCH

Clinical research is scientific research that involves humans as subjects. This type of research is most commonly seen in clinical pharmaceutical trials, which test potential new drugs and treatments on humans to check for both efficacy and safety. The research question no longer is, "How does this compound interact with cancer cells?" nor even "Can this compound possibly block the growth of cancer cells?" but "Is this compound safe and useful enough to give to cancer patients?"

Clinical research may also examine how behavior affects health. For example, a clinical researcher may examine how patient–provider communication affects birth control choice and usage.

PUBLIC HEALTH RESEARCH

Public health research focuses on the health of a population. It also tends to focus more on prevention and wellness than other types of research. Public health research encompasses many disciplines including:

- **Epidemiology:** Uses statistics about a population to investigate the relationship between exposure or experience and disease processes (e.g., smoking and lung cancer).
- **Biostatistics:** The study design, data collection, and analysis processes of studies focused on living organisms (e.g., collecting and analyzing data about smokers and lung cancer).

Another important subset is health services research, which focuses on the effectiveness of health systems, institutions, and delivery models and their resulting effects on cost, access, quality, and health outcomes. Examples may include examining how adopting electronic health records changes nursing behaviors, how the availability of generic drugs affects the treatment of uninsured patients, and what practices most reduce hospital-acquired infections.

You can think of these types of research as moving from looking at the trees (or even at the cells in a single leaf) to looking at the forest.

Institutions and Funding

Scientists perform research at a variety of public and private institutions. Funding for their activities may be provided by their own institution or by an outside group. Many for-profit corporations and government agencies keep everything in-house, employing scientists and funding their research. Things get more complex when more than one institution is involved; for example, a single scientist employed at a public university may pursue a project that draws on funding from the federal government, a nonprofit organization, the host university, and private industry. Let's discuss the major players in the research world.

ACADEMIC

A large percentage of research scientists are employed by universities and medical colleges, where they educate students as well as conduct research. However, only 20% of research and development (R&D) completed at academic centers is funded by the host institution; the remainder is provided by federal, state, and local governments, private foundations, and industry.[2]

PUBLIC

Federal, state, and local government agencies are involved in all areas of the research process. Most medical research falls under the federal Department of Health & Human Services (HHS), which controls the National Institutes of Health (NIH), along with agencies that focus on health services research (Agency for Health Research and Quality), basic research (National Science Foundation), and public health research (Centers for Disease Control and Prevention), among others. A variety of other federal agencies participate in research, including the Department of Defense and the National Institute of Food and Agriculture. Each of these agencies employs its own researchers as well as funds projects at other institutions. The NIH alone has nearly 6,000 scientists on staff and provides grant funding for another 300,000 researchers at outside institutions.[3]

INDUSTRY

Pharmaceutical, biotechnology, and medical technology companies often conduct research in their own organizations, with their own employees and labs. They also fund research at academic institutions.

PRIVATE NONPROFIT

Private nonprofit organizations in the research field usually fund outside scientists using a grant system similar to that of the NIH. However, some conduct research in-house as well. One example is the RAND Corporation, a relatively small organization that conducts health services research. An example of a much larger organization is the World Health Organization (WHO), part of the United Nations, which conducts public health research globally.

FUNDING

Research accounts for 2% of the total spending on health care in the U.S.[4] Here are the top funders of health research in 2012, according to the research advocacy group Research!America:[5]

Source	Funds
Industry	
Pharmaceutical R&D	$36,810 million
Biotechnology R&D	$19,300M
Medical Technology R&D	$13,059M
Federal Government	
National Institutes of Health	$30,012M
Department of Defense	$2,412M
National Science Foundation	$2,075M

Source	Funds
Federal Government *(continued)*	
Department of Agriculture	$1,953M
Department of Energy	$1,020M
Department of Veterans Affairs	$580M
Environmental Protection Agency	$568M
National Institute of Standards and Technology	$557M
Centers for Disease Control and Prevention	$408M
Food and Drug Administration	$406M
Others	$1,025M
Other Sources	
Universities (Institutional Funds)	$12,445M
State and Local Governments	$3,819M
Independent Research Institutes	$1,538M
Philanthropic Foundations	$1,322M
Voluntary Health Associations	$1,074M
Total	$130 billion

Research!America, "2010 U.S. Investment in Health Research,"
August 2011.

The "Sequester" and Decreased Research Funding

In March 2013, budget cuts that Congress mandated in 2011—collectively known as the "sequester"—started taking effect. The sequester cuts a total of $85.3 billion, spread among various departments, including defense, Medicare, and, of interest for this chapter, the NIH.[6] The NIH's budget was cut by 5%, or $1.5 billion.[7] Accordingly, the NIH approved 703 fewer grants in 2013 than in 2012,[8] and Research!America estimates the decline in funding will cost "20,500 jobs nationwide, and $3 billion in economic activity."[7]

Typically, much academic medical research is conducted at universities, to the tune of $30 billion of federal funding each year[9] (though that isn't limited to medical research). Since the cuts took effect in 2013, universities

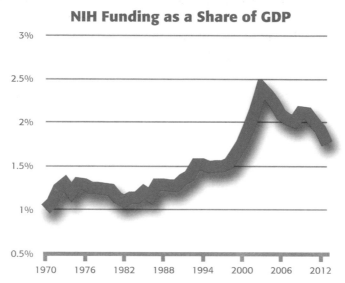

NIH Funding as a Share of GDP

Kwame Boadi, "Erosion of Funding for the National Institutes of Health Threatens U.S. Leadership in Biomedical Research," March 2014.

are reporting a reduction in graduate student admissions and cancellations of ongoing projects.[10]

The funding cuts cause both short-term and long-term concerns. Short-term, the cuts have forced many labs to cut staff and even to close.[8] Long-term, the cuts may discourage students from pursuing medical research, either heading to industry or leaving science altogether, causing a "brain drain," which could decrease the productivity of medical research for years to come.[11]

The Research and Development Process

The process starts when researchers apply for grant funding, among stiff competition. Funded grants reward research focused on new discoveries. Researchers spend months to years on this research, the outcomes of which are kept private unless and until the researchers publish their findings. Today, more than 20,000 active scientific journals publish 1.35 million articles each year.[12] Next, industry identifies a tiny fraction of promising findings for drug and device development and chooses directions for manufacturing, some of which are fruitful while others are not. Once a drug or device is created, it undergoes an approval process by the FDA.

There are several bottlenecks to note in the process: what gets funded, what gets published, what gets picked up by drug manufacturers, what passes clinical trials, what gets approved by the government, and, finally, what is found to be clinically useful.

The Medical Research and Development Pipeline

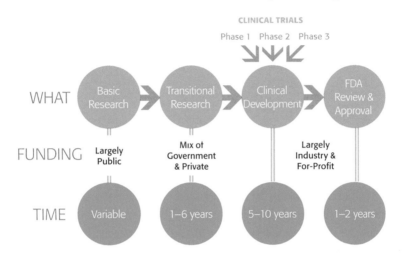

Adapted from: *National Center for Advancing Translational Sciences, "Why Translational Research Matters," June 2013.* Used with permission.

PEER REVIEW SYSTEM

Medical peer review encompasses both scientific research and clinical behavior. Articles submitted to scientific journals are judged by a committee comprising researchers whose expertise is in the same field. Each reviewer is given an advance copy of the article and may accept it as is, request revisions, or reject the article. Reviewers are expected to recuse themselves if they are working on the same project or cannot provide an objective analysis, so that conflict of interest will not bias the review.

Peer review is also used in clinical practice. Hospital discipline committees and expert witnesses at medical malpractice trials employ peer review to judge physicians' decisions. Who makes up the "peers" varies by situation and institution, but health professionals are usually evaluated by other members of their discipline (e.g., physical therapy) and specialty (e.g., cardiology).

Peer review works well because scientific practice and research are judged by others in the field—peers—who have a greater understanding of the material than the lay public, but it's not a perfect system. In research, the veracity of the data is assumed (thus, the system is not designed to detect fraud). Scientists are often asked to objectively judge the work of their competitors. In clinical practice, the physicians who make up discipline committees are often co-workers; the physician you are judging today may be judging you next week. Such practices can lead to leniency rather than rigorous challenges.

REGULATION AND OVERSIGHT

Depending on the type of research and how it's funded, research may be regulated by the government, the institution where it's being conducted, or both. Let's look at some of the regulators and ethical principles more closely.

Office of Research Integrity (ORI): This is a branch of the federal Department of Health & Human Services, charged by Congress with maintaining regulatory oversight on research. It regulates all research except that subject to the FDA (U.S. Food and Drug Administration). ORI monitors institutional investigations of research misconduct and reviews policies involving such misconduct.[13]

Institutional Review Boards (IRB): These peer review bodies of medical professionals, often multidisciplinary, are charged with protecting the safety and welfare of human subjects in medical research and clinical trials. IRBs focus primarily on protecting potential research subjects and must approve protocols, consent forms, etc. You'll find these at every institution that conducts medical research; all research that involves humans (even if only collecting data from their medical records) requires approval from an IRB. IRBs are required to have at least one nonscientist member and at least one member unaffiliated with the research institution.

Health Insurance Portability and Accountability Act (HIPAA): If you work in the health professions, you will most certainly have to learn more about HIPAA, which enacted the first universal code in the U.S. to protect patient privacy. HIPAA protects patient confidentiality and informed consent, regulating how patients' personal health information can be viewed, stored, and used in both clinical care and in research. It also contains a multitude of regulations that have increased the time and cost for many research studies. (See Chapter 3 for more information.)

Research Is Important for Health

In this chapter, we want you to learn about some of the issues troubling the research system, including questions of validity and news of funding cuts. We also want you to learn how important research is to improving health. Evidence indicates that roughly 50% of longevity gains in the past century can be attributed to medical care.[14] The medical research system has built and bolstered that care. David Cutler, a Harvard economist, gives an idea of the value of medical research by focusing on cardiovascular disease, the number one cause of death.[15]

Cutler tells us (a) that research in cardiovascular disease has produced high tech innovation, low tech innovation, and behavioral changes causing health improvements; (b) that such health improvements have increased average life expectancy by 4.5 years; and (c) that the amount of research dollars spent for longevity gain means funding research is a steal. To quote:

> "The average 45 year old spends about $30,000 more currently on cardiovascular disease than he or she did in 1950. But the gains from longer life are much greater. Using common values in the literature, we estimate that the improved health resulting from medical treatment changes is approximately $120,000. The rate of return to medical technology innovation is therefore about 4 to 1. The return to new knowledge is even greater. We estimate that basic knowledge about disease risk has a return of about 30 to 1."[15]

But there's more to life than death, and medical research has been similarly important for improving quality of life. Imagine also the rate of return for research that allows us to remove cataracts, reduce post-surgical pain, treat heartburn, and replace worn-down joints. Looking to the future, developing fields such as stem-cell therapy and genomics may lead to even greater improvements in quality and quantity of life.

Pharmaceuticals

A pharmaceutical is a chemical substance used to prevent, treat, or cure a disease. In the 1920s, there weren't many drugs beyond aspirin, codeine, morphine, digitalis, nitroglycerin, quinine, and insulin. Today, more than 10,000 prescription drugs available in the U.S.[16] represent a $260 billion industry.[17] The average American fills more than 12 prescriptions per year.[18] (Although, interestingly, one-third of all prescriptions written by providers are never filled by patients![19])

Pharmaceuticals are usually divided into two groups:

1. **Small molecule drugs** are chemically synthesized molecules sometimes derived from naturally occurring products. Most prescription drugs available, from Valium to Vicodin to Viagra, are small molecule drugs.
2. **Large molecule drugs,** also known as "biologics," are produced by living cells rather than through chemical synthesis. They're larger and more complex than small molecule pharmaceuticals and, not surprisingly, usually cost a whole lot more. Examples of biologics include insulin, vaccines, and the anti-cancer drug Avastin.

The Industry

So far, we've talked about research in terms of intellectual inquiry and the social good, which seems quite lofty and academic. However, treatment—and research—is also a business. Pharmaceutical companies invest lots of money in R&D to identify, develop, and test potential therapeutics, and they're heavily regulated by the government. Don't feel too bad for them, though, as they end up with quite a nice financial reward from the drugs that do make it to market.

The five largest pharmaceutical companies, by revenue[20] are:

Company	Country	Annual Revenues	Employees	Top Seller
Pfizer	USA	$58.9 billion	100,800	Lyrica
Novartis	SWI	$56.7B	120,000	Gleevec
Merck	USA	$47.3B	83,000	Januvia
Sanofi	FRA	$44.9B	111,974	Lantus
GlaxoSmithKline	UK	$41.9B	99,488	Advair

Critics of the pharmaceutical industry call it "Big Pharma." Because this is a biased term, we won't use it, but it's easy to see why people might use the term for the industry.

Government Regulation

The mission of the FDA is to regulate and ensure the safety of goods affecting individual and public health, including food and nutritional supplements, drugs, vaccines and biotechnology, radiation-emitting devices, cosmetics, tobacco products, and veterinary products. To give an idea of its scope, the FDA regulates about 25% of all consumer goods sold in the U.S.[21] However, it approves very few pharmaceuticals—for example, only 27 new drugs passed muster in 2013.[22]

The path to approval for a new pharmaceutical agent is long and stringent. A manufacturer can apply for a new drug if it's a "new molecular entity" or a previously used molecular entity employed in a new way. The FDA requires several stages of clinical testing before allowing a new drug on the market; each stage adds more data about efficacy and safety. The entire process looks something like this:

1. A pharmaceutical company identifies a promising molecular compound. Testing begins on individual cells, and, if successful, proceeds to testing on live animals. The company can then submit an **Investigational New Drug (IND)** application to the FDA. The FDA has 30 days to review the IND, and, if approved, trials on human subjects can begin.

2. **Phase I:** The drug is tested on a small group (20–100) of healthy volunteers to make sure it's not immediately toxic and to determine some basic information about how the drug is absorbed and excreted from the body.

3. **Phase II:** The drug is tested on a larger group (30–300) of volunteers, all with the disease the drug targets (e.g., diabetes for insulin). This phase continues the experiments from Phase I and starts to assess the drug's safety and efficacy at different doses.

4. **Phase III:** Randomized controlled trials, usually double-blinded and multicenter, sometimes compared with a competitor, of a large group (300–3,000) of patients with the disease of interest. Half of the patients receive the new drug and half receive a placebo or current gold-standard treatment. After a sufficient amount of time, the

outcomes of the two groups are compared. Phase III trials are the most expensive and time-consuming part of the approvals process.

5. The manufacturer submits a **New Drug Application (NDA)** to the FDA, which contains all information known about the drug, both negative and positive, in all circumstances.

6. The FDA has 10 months to review the application. It may approve it, approve it on condition of Phase IV trials, or reject the application. Once the FDA has approved an NDA, the drug may be sold immediately.

7. **Phase IV:** Post-approval monitoring of a group of patients on the drug to determine side effects and drug interactions.

8. For every drug approved, the manufacturer is required to collect reports of adverse events and drug interactions and submit them in periodic reports to the FDA.[23]

Several variations to be aware of include[a]:

▸ **Treatment IND:** This is an exception to the typical NDA process that the FDA uses to make promising new drugs available to desperately ill patients even before the drug has been formally approved.

▸ **Supplemental NDA:** After a drug is approved, if the manufacturer wishes to change the dose, strength, manufacturing process, or labeling, it must submit a supplemental NDA. This is the pathway by which drugs are approved for new indications and for pediatric patients, both of which require new clinical trials.

▸ **Abbreviated NDA:** This is the pathway used for approval of a generic version of an already approved medication. It's faster and cheaper than a typical NDA because the molecular compound had already proven safe and efficacious in the original application.

▸ **Orphan drugs:** To stimulate research into rare diseases, the federal government gives special incentives to "orphan drugs," whose potential market is less than 200,000 individuals. These incentives include tax credits, expedited reviews, research grants, market exclusivity, and fee exemptions.

Intellectual Property

A new drug, like any other invention, receives intellectual property (IP) protection from the U.S. government, which is achieved in two ways:

---

a   There are also a number of new pathways for expedited FDA approval, including Fast Track, Breakthrough Therapy, Accelerated Approval, and Priority Review.[75]

1. **Patents:** Many aspects of a pharmaceutical can be patented, including the molecular structure, method of use, and manufacturing process. These patents last for 20 years, but most drugs are patented early in development, years before the FDA approves them. The duration of a patent on a new drug can be extended by up to five years to compensate for time lost to clinical trials and FDA review. By the time a drug is released to market, it typically has eight to 14 years of patent protection left.

2. **Data Exclusivity:** For a period of time after a new drug is approved, the safety and efficacy data from its clinical trials cannot be used by generic manufacturers. Small molecule drugs have data exclusivity for five to seven-and-a-half years after approval while biologics have 12 years. Data exclusivity can be extended by filing a supplemental NDA for a new indication (adding three years[b]) or a pediatric indication (adding six months).

An FDA-approved drug represents a culmination of years of research, development, and clinical trials—not to mention hundreds of millions of dollars. IP protection is meant to ensure that the drug is protected from competition for some time, allowing the manufacturer to recoup its investment. However, finding the right duration for patent protection and data exclusivity is tricky: Longer IP protection keeps low-cost generics off the market, translating to higher prices for patients and insurers, while a shorter duration would decrease the financial reward for the manufacturer and reduce the incentive to develop new drugs in the future.

Generics and Biosimilars

After the patent for a small molecule drug has expired,[c] other manufacturers can make their own version of the same molecule; these are dubbed "generic" pharmaceuticals. Generic manufacturers must conduct trials to show that their version of the drug is absorbed and distributed in the body in the same way as the original, "brand-name" drug—that it is "bioequivalent." If bioequivalence is proven, the generic can be approved via the

---

b   Not available for biologics.
c   There are *many* more legal issues, but we'll just mention one important point: Four years after a new small molecule drug is approved, any other manufacturer can file a lawsuit claiming that the drug's patents are invalid. If the court agrees, the company that filed suit is allowed to start making generics immediately. Take-home message: Patent protection for new, small molecule drugs may be cut off after four years due to legal challenges.

Abbreviated NDA pathway and sold openly on the marketplace alongside the original drug. Generic drugs are much cheaper than brand-name drugs because generic manufacturers don't have to invest in research, development, testing, or marketing pharmaceuticals. In several states, pharmacies can automatically substitute a generic for any bioequivalent prescription unless the provider or patient specifically requests the brand-name drug. Today, 84% of all prescriptions are written for generics.[24]

The generic version of a biologic drug is known as a "biosimilar." Biosimilars are much more difficult to create than generics because the manufacturing and purification process for biologics is far more complex than for small molecule drugs. Nevertheless, the ACA (Affordable Care Act) mandates a process for the FDA to approve and regulate biosimilars, so expect to see more on the market in the next decade.

Payment and PBMs

The way pharmaceuticals are paid for in the U.S. is similar to the general health care payment systems outlined in Chapter 2 with a few extra layers of complexity thrown on top for good measure. Two terms you'll need to know: A **formulary** is a list of the prescription drugs approved for use in a health care institution or a health plan, and a **pharmacy benefits manager (PBM)** is a for-profit company that manages pharmaceutical sales for a health care plan. Pharmaceutical delivery and payment differ significantly in the inpatient and outpatient settings.

In the hospital, the formulary is regulated by the hospital's Pharmacy & Therapeutics (P&T) committee. Drugs approved by the P&T committee are purchased and stocked by the hospital pharmacy. Providers may prescribe any drug on formulary for a patient while she or he is in the hospital. These drugs aren't billed separately but are bundled into the price for the entire episode of care, as with a Diagnosis-Related Group (DRG, page 50).

Outside the hospital, most insurance plans contract with PBMs to handle outpatient pharmaceuticals for their beneficiaries. PBMs negotiate drug prices, purchase drugs from pharmaceutical manufacturers, and manage the distribution of those drugs to patients, either through contracts with retail pharmacies (e.g., Walgreens) or via their own mail-order pharmacies. Formularies for outpatient medicines are established by PBMs and/or insurance plans. In contrast to hospital formularies, these lists indicate how much a patient will have to contribute as a co-payment for any approved drug. PBMs and insurance plans try to keep their costs low by steering patients to generics and other cheaper drugs, so they set lower patient co-payments; this system of classifying drugs by co-pay is known as a "tiered formulary." In a typical plan, a generic statin prescription requires $10 patient co-pay (tier 1) while the co-pay for Crestor, a brand-name statin, is $40 (tier 3). The largest PBM is Express Scripts.

Pharmaceuticals and payments are shuffled between manufacturers, pharmacies, hospitals, wholesalers, PBMs, private insurers, government programs, third-party administrators, patient assistance programs, employers, and, finally, patients.[25] As you might imagine, any system this complex has many issues. In one all-too-common scenario, a sick patient is hospitalized and his or her physicians start the patient on several different medicines to control the disease and symptoms. Over the course of a week, the dosages and formulations of the medicines are adjusted until a good regimen is found, and the patient is well enough to go home. Sounds simple enough, until you remember that the patient's inpatient formulary (determined by the hospital) and outpatient formulary (tiered, determined by the PBM) are different. So, at discharge, the patient's prescriptions have to be switched, and he or she goes home on a completely different medication regimen, which may or may not work. This example is another reminder that the way the U.S. health care system is structured and funded—although it may seem abstract and removed from day-to-day clinical care—can, and often does, directly impact patients' health.

Medical Devices

Pharmaceuticals and medical devices are both real-world applications of research. Medical devices can improve health and treatment through:
  ▸ Better diagnostics (e.g., CT scans)
  ▸ Safer and less invasive procedures (e.g., laparoscopic surgery)
  ▸ Longer lives (e.g., pacemakers)
  ▸ Easier lives (e.g., full joint replacements)
The number and complexity of available medical devices have increased significantly over the past 25 years. Today, more than $150 billion is spent on medical devices in the country each year.[26]

The Industry

The U.S. has the world's largest medical device industry. The five companies with the greatest revenues are:[27]

Company	Country	Annual Revenues	Employees
Johnson & Johnson	USA	$27.4 billion	127,600
GE Healthcare	USA	$18.3B	54,000
Siemens Healthcare	GER	$17.5B	51,000
Medtronic	USA	$16.2B	45,000
Baxter	USA	$14.2B	51,000

Government Regulation

The FDA regulates the approval and sales of medical devices in the U.S. The specifics of the approval process for each device depend on the level of risk to the patient. The FDA categorizes every device as low (Class I), intermediate (Class II), or high risk (Class III), and the requirements to prove safety and effectiveness vary accordingly. This makes sense—complicated, high-risk devices such as pacemakers ought to go through more testing than simple, low-risk devices such as tongue depressors. The FDA can approve new devices in one of three ways:[28]

1. **Registration:** Class I and low-risk Class II devices don't have to undergo a true approval process. Manufacturers of these products simply have to register new devices with the FDA when they enter the market.

2. **Substantial Equivalence/510(k):** Intermediate-risk Class II devices that can demonstrate "substantial equivalence" to an FDA-approved medical device already on the market, are cleared by the 510(k) process. Substantial equivalence originally referred to new versions of previously approved devices with minor modifications, but the 510(k) pathway also is now used for new devices with a similar intended use and safety profile as a previously approved product, even if the new device has a different mechanism of action and/or is constructed of different materials.[29] Randomized clinical trials aren't usually required for the 510(k) process. More than 3,000 products are approved by this pathway each year.[30]

3. **Premarket Approval:** Class III devices are approved by the FDA via a process known as a Premarket Approval (PMA), which is similar to the

method used for new pharmaceuticals. Clinical trials demonstrating safety and efficacy of the new product are required before the device can be approved through the PMA pathway. This process is much more expensive and time-consuming than the 510(k) pathway. The FDA approves fewer than 50 devices by the PMA pathway each year. [31]

The FDA also maintains a system for tracking adverse events for products approved and released into the market. Manufacturers are required to report to the FDA any serious device-related adverse events that caused or could have caused serious injury or death. Similar requirements exist for hospitals and other health care facilities. The FDA receives tens of thousands of these reports each year.[32] After receiving reports about a specific device, the FDA has a range of options, from further study to mandatory recall. The FDA recalled 1,190 medical devices models in 2012, including 57 defective devices—like fracture-prone pacemaker wires—with a "reasonable probability" of causing serious adverse outcomes or death.[33,34]

The Affordable Care Act also enacted a new excise tax of 2.3% for medical devices.[35] See Chapter 5 for more details.

Issues

These issues are complicated and deep: The more you learn, the more shades of nuance appear. We can't fully explore the issues here, but we'll introduce some major issues facing these vitally important industries. (See Suggested Reading at the end of the book if you would like to explore them in more depth.)

Utility of Research Findings

PLACEBO EFFECT

A common way for a new drug to be approved by the FDA is to prove that it leads to a statistically significant health improvement over a placebo. A placebo is a medical treatment that has no direct physiological effect; i.e., a sham treatment. The effect of a placebo is psychological, though studies show that the psychological can become the physiological.

Placebo drugs may be active (such as antibiotics given for a viral infection) or inactive (such as a sugar pill). Placebos also may be sham surgeries (some of the most effective placebos!) or clinically unrelated procedures (such as sham acupuncture). In addition, the physician–patient relationship itself may even establish a placebo effect. The placebo effect can work even when patients know they're receiving a placebo.

The placebo effect is a mixture of expectations and conditioning,[36] the idea being that people experience what they expect to (whether positive or negative—a "nocebo"). This effect isn't just theoretical; in fact, it's real and surprisingly large. For example, placebos are an effective treatment for 32% of patients with depression (compared to 48% for SSRIs, the most popular type of antidepressants[37]). And, weird but true, the placebo effect seems to be growing more potent over time.[38] As you can imagine, the placebo effect is a major concern for those involved in developing new drugs.

VALIDITY CONCERNS

Scientific research is susceptible to many problems:
▸ Researchers may frame their questions in a way that points to predetermined conclusions.
▸ They may choose a poorly representative population sample.
▸ They may make a mistake in data analysis.
▸ A journal may publish or reject articles for reasons other than the validity of the science.
▸ The media may report conclusions that weren't truly there.
▸ The study may be invalidated later but never retracted in the eyes of other researchers and the public.

Further, science barrels forward, and studies may quickly go out of date as new methods and materials are introduced. No matter how exacting and hard-working scientists may be, there's no perfect research study. Thus, a growing number of scientists have begun to analyze not only biomedical questions, but also the research world itself and how it's affected by the problems listed. Some of their findings are startling:
▸ Many studies are refuted at a later date. Of the 49 most influential studies during a 13-year period, 45 of them found an intervention to be effective. Of those 45, 32% have subsequently been shown to be wrong or exaggerated.[39,40]

▸ Researchers are more likely to submit, and journals are more likely to publish, experiments with positive results,[41,42] termed "publication bias." Five identical experiments may only produce the desired result once; but if that one trial is the only one submitted and published, the general public would have the false impression that 100% of the experiments were successful.[d]

▸ Conflict of interest may arise. New medical and pharmaceutical products are subject to multiple trials to prove efficacy and safety. Yet many of these studies are funded by the very same company that produces the product. Not surprisingly, trials funded by a private company are more likely—four times as much, in one major study[43]—to have results that benefit the sponsoring company than are trials funded by others.

▸ The research system lacks a consistent way to retract published research later determined to be invalid. Researchers often continue to cite the results of invalid papers for many years after they have been retracted; even more surprising, many papers found to be fraudulent are never retracted at all.[44]

You may argue with any of these claims. However, they are generally accepted and lauded within the research community; we present them here as the contrarian view of established practices.

Wouldn't it be something if this research got refuted someday, though?

Evidence-Based Medicine and Clinical Practice Guidelines

Evidence-based medicine (EBM) seeks to integrate the best research evidence with clinical judgment and the patient's values and preferences, while keeping in mind safety, effectiveness, and the cost of medical procedures. Although this idea seems rather obvious—basing medical decisions on the best possible evidence—the commitment to using EBM is relatively new.

EBM isn't intended to be formulaic; proponents emphasize that EBM practice does not rely solely on research evidence, nor historical precedent or anecdote, but combines them with bedside experience and with the goals for a

---

d To counteract publication bias, the NIH has created a publicly available trial registry at www. ClinicalTrials.Gov. There, researchers can prospectively catalog their trials and report basic results after completion, even if the research isn't published in a journal. The FDA and several consortiums of medical journals now require many trials to be registered at ClinicalTrials.Gov.

patient's care. The danger comes from providers who put too much focus on research findings without considering them within the clinical context.

One widespread application of EBM to everyday clinical care is the Clinical Practice Guideline (CPG). CPGs serve as reference guides for what the best available evidence indicates health care providers should do in a given situation. All providers will consult some practice guidelines during their careers. One well-known example of a CPG is the Ottawa Ankle Rules. These guidelines help physicians determine whether an X-ray should be taken for ankle and foot injuries based on a patient's symptoms. Yet, despite the utility of CPGs (the Ottawa Ankle Rules are correct for

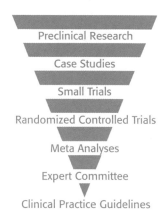

Preclinical Research

Case Studies

Small Trials

Randomized Controlled Trials

Meta Analyses

Expert Committee

Clinical Practice Guidelines

nearly all ankle and foot injuries and can reduce the number of unnecessary X-rays by at least one-third[45]), not all physicians use them all the time. Fewer than one-third of American emergency physicians use the Ottawa Ankle Rules most of the time;[46] in general, a recent study found only 55% of Americans who visited a physician received the recommended care based on available guidelines.[47]

Why don't clinicians use clinical practice guidelines more often? As with many topics we cover in this book, translating the theoretical benefits of EBM to the real world is much more difficult than it would seem at first glance. Many health care professionals have expressed deep-seated concerns about CPGs, and with EBM in general. Some of their concerns include:

▸ EBM is based on evidence from clinical trials that may be less relevant than you'd think. Clinical trials often focus on a select patient population (e.g., healthy females between 18–50 in Sweden) that may not apply to a given patient. They also usually compare two treatments for a medical condition when, in reality, a range of options are available; and practical considerations like cost and access aren't usually included.

▸ CPGs focus too much on the "average" patient, so guidelines aren't applicable to patients with unique characteristics or multiple medical conditions. Conversely, creating different CPGs for every conceivable case would be expensive and make it impossible for physicians to wade through them all.

▸ One of the key tools of EBM is the meta-analysis, which combines data from many different clinical trials. Pooling data is intended to make the resulting conclusions more robust, but a meta-analysis is only as good— or as up-to-date—as the trials it draws from. Further, meta-analyses of the same data can come to different conclusions depending on their design and inclusion criteria, so bias among the designers of the meta-analysis is highly important but often overlooked.

▸ Requiring providers to follow guidelines erodes clinical autonomy. Many health professionals feel that "cookbook medicine," as some derisively refer to EBM, underestimates the value of personal judgment gained from years of clinical practice, instead leading providers to make decisions according to a rule rather than responding to the needs of the individual patient.[48]

▸ There is still no consistent method for highlighting studies weakened by conflict of interest or bias.

▸ Many different organizations create CPGs, and multiple guidelines may be available for the same condition. Unfortunately, they often disagree. For example, the American Congress of Obstetrics and Gynecology guidelines recommend routine mammography to screen for breast cancer every one to two years for women age 40–49 years,[49] while the federal U.S. Preventive Services Task Force instead recommends starting routine mammography at age 50.[50]

In short, evidence-based medicine and clinical practice guidelines are key developments in modern medicine that show promise for significant improvements in health care quality. However, substantial barriers exist to the widespread application of EBM to everyday clinical practice. Furthermore, the elephant in the room is that the utility of EBM is limited by how much we still don't know about medicine and the human body. Consider just how many diseases are "idiopathic"—a fancy term for "we have no clue."[e]

SIGNIFICANCE: STATISTICAL VS. CLINICAL

To be approved by the FDA, a new drug must prove to be significantly more efficacious than placebo or the current gold-standard treatment in clinical trials. What constitutes a "significant" improvement is determined by sophisticated statistical methods. However, statistically significant improvement may

---

e   Or, as the old joke goes, an idiopathic disease is one in which the doctor is an idiot and the patient is pathetic.

be as small as 1%, which may not be clinically meaningful in a "real world" treatment setting. By contrast, the United Kingdom's National Institute for Health and Clinical Excellence emphasizes clinical significance and cost-effectiveness, rather than statistical significance, which assesses the practical relevance of the finding. Aside from the technical definitions for both statistical and clinical significance, there's the meta-question of what level of significance should be necessary for physicians to prescribe drugs for patients who must pay for them and who may experience side effects.

Government Regulation

Many criticize the way the government, specifically the FDA, regulates the pharmaceutical and medical device industries. Here we list some of the most common arguments regarding government regulations. As with other areas of the book we aren't endorsing any specific opinion but want the reader to be familiar with the range of views.

TOO MUCH REGULATION

- The FDA approvals process for drugs and devices is too expensive. The cost to develop and test a new drug and bring it to market now exceeds a billion dollars,[51] and these astronomical expenses translate to higher prices for consumers.
- The FDA approvals process is too long, which keeps patients waiting for desperately needed treatments. The FDA trial and approval process for a new cancer drug, for instance, usually takes more than five years.[52]
- The FDA approvals process is too rigorous, so drug and device companies cut back on their R&D spending because of the low probability that new drugs will actually make it to the market.
- The approvals process in the European Union is easier and quicker than in the U.S.[53] Manufacturers may simply avoid the FDA approvals process, leading to medical devices and medications that are available in many other countries but not in the U.S.[54]

NOT ENOUGH REGULATION

- The FDA prefers two Phase III trials that show a new drug is efficacious before approval; however, a company can run as many

Phase III trials as it needs to get those two. A drug can be ineffective in eight out of 10 trials and still be approved by the FDA. These negative results are viewed as proprietary and are kept confidential by the FDA.[55]

▸ Clinical trials of new drugs and devices are too short, and many new products are released to the market without a good understanding of their long-term adverse effects.

▸ The FDA approves new pharmaceuticals for specific medical indications, but once a drug is released to the market it may be prescribed for any use. Most of these "off-label" prescriptions haven't been proven to be clinically effective. For example, gabapentin (Neurontin) is FDA-approved for the treatment of epilepsy and post-herpetic neuralgia, but more than 80% of nationwide gabapentin prescriptions are for other conditions, from hot flashes to restless leg syndrome.[56]

▸ Dietary supplements like vitamins and herbal therapies don't have to demonstrate safety or effectiveness before they are marketed and sold; in fact, the burden of proof is on the FDA to prove a product is unsafe before it has to be pulled from the market.

TOO MUCH INDUSTRY INFLUENCE

In 1992, Congress passed legislation, the Prescription Drug User Fee Act (known by the charming acronym PDUFA), to speed up the FDA drug approvals process. This legislation set specific deadlines for the FDA reviews of new pharmaceuticals. To pay for the extra staff needed to meet these deadlines, PDUFA also mandated a fee system for pharmaceutical companies that submit drugs for FDA review. Although PDUFA did succeed in significantly reducing the amount of time that drugs spend in the approvals process, it also has generated a tremendous amount of controversy. Fees paid by pharmaceutical companies now account for 70% of the FDA budget for drug review,[57] meaning, essentially, that the FDA is funded by the industry that it regulates. Similar legislation for the medical device industry (called MDUFMA, naturally) was enacted in 2002. It's beyond the scope of this book to determine if PDUFA and MDUFMA have led to worse health outcomes for patients, but the current set-up creates at least the appearance that the FDA has a major conflict of interest in regard to drug and device regulation.

Why Are Drug Prices So High?

This is a simple question with a very complicated—and only partially explainable—answer. We should be wary of over-simplification, as the situation is complex, but we'll try our best to break it down. First, some background:

Drug Prices in the U.S.: Drug pricing runs the gamut from $48 per year for generics at Walmart to $2,615 per year for the common cholesterol drug Crestor[58] to nearly $500,000 per year for Soliris, which treats paroxysmal nocturnal hemoglobinuria.[59] Even for the same drug, prices can vary over 400% when you shop around.[60] Most patients are protected from the full price of drugs by insurance, but the uninsured and underinsured feel the full brunt of this pricing.

What Drugs Cost Elsewhere: The U.S. spends far more than any other industrialized country on pharmaceuticals.

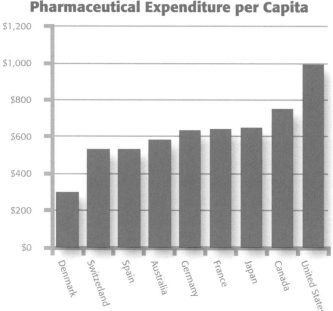

Pharmaceutical Expenditure per Capita

Organisation for Economic Co-operation and Development, "Health: Key Tables from OECD," Oct. 2013. Note: Expenditures in U.S. $ purchasing power parity. Data from 2010 and 2011.

Other industrialized countries are able to keep drug prices lower for patients by negotiating lower prices with manufacturers and regulating price-setting by industry. Some countries, like the UK, only pay for drugs that they determine to be clinically- and cost-effective. In the U.S., some pharmacy benefits managers, insurance plans, and government programs such as the VA negotiate with drug companies, but none has the market share to negotiate prices as low as a nationwide system can. However, in other countries, just as in the U.S., the justification for price-setting is not always transparent.[61]

Now, let's discuss the reasons for high drug prices in the U.S.

REASON #1: RESEARCH AND DEVELOPMENT COSTS ARE HIGH

To get a new drug on the market, companies must fund or find basic science research, fund continued research on what actually seems to be useful, apply for a patent, go through FDA approval, and, finally, manufacture and sell the drug. Very little of what goes into the first step (basic science) ends up in the last one (a sellable drug). So not only do you have to find a needle in a haystack, but then you have to make sure the needle won't hurt anyone and will actually sew before you can put it to work. These costs truly are enormous. To give you an idea:

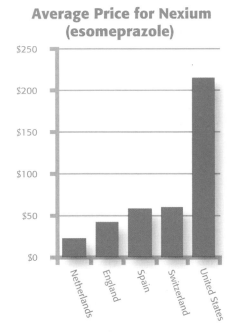

Average Price for Nexium (esomeprazole)

- In 2012, Merck spent $7.9 billion on R&D,[62] was issued 253 patents,[63] and had 96 prescription drugs on the market (total, not just those approved that year).[64,65]
- The average cost of developing a single drug is $1.2 billion, and only 1 in 5,000 compounds are successful.[66]
- Only 20% of medications brought to market make a profit.[66]

Clearly, R&D costs *a lot* and productivity has dropped over the past 10 years, further decreasing

International Federation of Health Plans, "2013 Comparative Price Report," April 2014.
Used with permission.

return on investment.[67] To recoup their high up-front costs, manufacturers charge a hefty price for their brand-name drugs in the few years before generics enter the market.

REASON #2: MARKETING COSTS ARE HIGH

To thrive in the highly competitive drug and device marketplace, manufacturers devote a significant portion of their budgets to marketing to providers and patients. One study estimated the total amount spent by drug companies for promotion in 2012 at $27 billion; 55% of the total was spent on detailing to physicians, 21% on drug samples, and 11% on direct-to-consumer advertising.[68] (Note that drug and device manufacturers introduced regulations in 2009 limiting their interactions with providers, including a prohibition on gift giving.)[69] Interestingly, the U.S. and New Zealand are the only two industrialized countries where direct-to-consumer advertising of pharmaceuticals is legal. As with any consumer product, advertising costs are high because they pay off.

REASON #3: WE HAVE NO IDEA

Even knowing what we know, how specific drug prices are set is often totally unclear. As with any capitalist system, prices are, to an extent, simply what the market will bear. Though we know that competition reduces costs, no one in the public knows the metrics used by drug manufacturers to set prices during patent periods.

Nexium, which treats heartburn, costs $295 in the U.S. but $23 in the Netherlands. Why is the U.S. price so much higher? Who knows! All we do know is that this is what the market will bear.

Some emphasize that drug prices are high because we're also paying for innovation—between 2000 and 2009, three-fifths of all drug patents worldwide came from the U.S.[70]—and that the high prices we pay subsidize the relatively low price of drugs in other countries. This raises several interesting questions:

- ▶ How much of the pharmaceutical business is truly innovative?
- ▶ How necessary is the U.S. intellectual property system to maintain that innovation?
- ▶ Can we reduce America's subsidization of other countries' drug prices without losing pharmaceutical jobs and investment money to

international competitors?

‣ To what extent should we be willing to trade access for innovation, or vice versa?

‣ To what extent can we solve the access problem without driving health care costs up even more?

Trying to answer any of these questions breeds even more perplexing questions—each topic can fill (and has!) entire books. Please see Suggested Reading to learn more.

Intersections and Conflicts of Interest

As we've discussed, the research, pharmaceutical, and device worlds intersect, interact, and overlap. Any time you have an intermingling of groups with diverse motivations—mixed with billions of dollars—conflicts of interest are bound to arise. Medical research is no exception. Scientific researchers investigating a new drug or device are often funded by the very same company that makes and sells said product. Pharmaceutical and device companies pay health care providers and researchers to participate in speakers' bureaus and conferences and to consult about new products. Many post-graduate fellowships are funded by industry. More than 72,000 pharmaceutical sales representatives are employed to visit physicians' offices to market drugs and distribute free samples.[71]

It should be no surprise, then, that according to a survey in 2007, 94% of physicians reported some kind of connection to industry during the previous year.[72] The level of the relationship was affected by the type of specialty and practice. (For instance, family physicians and solo practitioners are more likely to meet with drug reps.)

Some of these relationships may even cross legal lines. In 2005, the federal government opened an investigation of the five largest hip and spine implant manufacturers for violation of anti-kickback laws. The government alleged that the "consulting" fees paid to some surgeons by device companies were little more than bribes for surgeons to use a specific product. The investigation was settled without any company admitting guilt, but the manufacturers did agree to pay a $310 million fine, instituted major changes to their business practices, and accepted strict federal oversight of their interactions with physicians.[73]

Publicity about conflicts of interest in medicine led to the Physician Payments Sunshine Act, a federal law passed in 2010. This act requires companies to report any gift or payment to a physician that is worth $10 or more. The federal government then posts the records of these payments[74] online for public review at the CMS Open Payments website.

While expensive dinners with drug reps may seem like an obvious conflict of interest deserving to be eradicated, interactions among physicians, researchers, professors, and industry are more subtle and more controversial. Clinicians have generated the ideas behind many of the important medical innovations over the past 25 years, but, as mentioned earlier, the journey from a good idea to an FDA-approved drug or device is long and expensive. Without support from private industry, many innovations would never have reached the market. Furthermore, many feel there's a lack of evidence to demonstrate that relationships between physicians, researchers, and industry actually lead to worse health outcomes for patients.

References

1. Dawkins R. To Live at All Is Miracle Enough. old.richarddawkins.net/articles/91-to-live-at-all-is-miracle-enough. Accessed May 30, 2014.
2. National Science Foundation. Survey of Research and Development Expenditures at Universities and Colleges. www.nsf.gov/statistics/srvyrdexpenditures/. Accessed June 28, 2014.
3. National Institutes of Health. NIH Budget. http://www.nih.gov/about/budget.htm. Accessed June 28, 2014.
4. Centers for Medicare & Medicaid Services. The Nation's Health Dollar ($2.8 Trillion), Calendar Year 2012: Where It Came From. www.cms.gov/Research-Statistics-Data-and-Systems/Statistics-Trends-and-Reports/NationalHealthExpendData/Downloads/PieChartSourcesExpenditures2012.pdf. Accessed June 15, 2014.
5. Research!America. Truth and Consequences: Health R&D Spending in the U.S. www.researchamerica.org/uploads/healthdollar12.pdf. Accessed June 28, 2014.
6. Matthews D. The Sequester: Absolutely Everything You Could Possibly Need to Know, in One FAQ. *The Washington Post.* Feb 20, 2013.
7. American Heart Association. Sequester Stories: How Heart and Stroke Research Hangs in the Balance. www.researchamerica.org/uploads/AHAbooklet.pdf. Accessed June 5, 2014.
8. Stratford M. As Effects of Sequester Take Effect, Scientists Worry About Future of Research. www.insidehighered.com/news/2013/09/09/effects-sequester-take-effect-scientists-worry-about-future-research#sthash.qCXMwfCV.dpbs. Accessed June 30, 2014.
9. Anderson N. Sequester Cuts University Research Funds. *The Washington Post.* March 17, 2013.
10. Anderson N. Universities Continue to Lobby against Sequester's Cuts of Research Funding. *The Washington Post.* Nov 12, 2013.
11. Firestone D. A Dark Future for Science. *The New York Times.* Sept 4, 2013.

12. Bjork BC, Roos A, et al. Scientific Journal Publishing: Yearly Volume and Open Access Availability. *Information Research.* 2009;14(1):391.

13. The Office of Research Integrity. About ORI. ori.hhs.gov/about/. Accessed July 2, 2014.

14. Cutler D, Rosen A, et al. The Value of Medical Spending in the United States, 1960–2000. *New England Journal of Medicine.* 2006(355):920.

15. Cutler D, Kadiyala S. The Return to Biomedical Research: Treatment and Behavioral Effects. citeseerx.ist.psu.edu/viewdoc/download?doi=10.1.1.200.7197&rep=rep1&type=pdf. Accessed June 5, 2014.

16. Institute for Safe Medication Practices. A Call to Action: Protecting U.S. Citizens from Inappropriate Medication Use. www.ismp.org/pressroom/viewpoints/CommunityPharmacy.pdf. Accessed June 5, 2014.

17. United States Census Bureau. The 2012 Statistical Abstract—Table 159. www.census.gov/compendia/statab/. Accessed July 1, 2014.

18. The Henry J. Kaiser Family Foundation. Retail Prescription Drugs Filled at Pharmacies (Annual Per Capita). kff.org/other/state-indicator/retail-rx-drugs-per-capita/. Accessed June 5, 2014.

19. Tamblyn R, Eguale T, et al. The Incidence and Determinants of Primary Nonadherence with Prescribed Medication in Primary Care: A Cohort Study. *Annals of Internal Medicine.* 2014/04/01 2014;160(7):441.

20. Contract Pharma. Top 20 Pharma Report: Our Annual Look at the 20 Biggest Players in the Pharmaceutical Marketplace. www.contractpharma.com/issues/2013-07/view_features/top-20-pharma-report-/. Accessed June 4, 2014.

21. Institute for International Economic Policy. U.S. Food and Drug Administration. www.gwu.edu/~iiep/governance/briefs/11FDA.pdf. Accessed June 28, 2014.

22. US Food and Drug Administration. Approved Drugs 2013. www.fda.gov/downloads/Drugs/DevelopmentApprovalProcess/DrugInnovation/UCM381803.pdf. Accessed June 4, 2014.

23. U.S. Food and Drug Administration. CFR - Code of Federal Regulations Title 21. www.accessdata.fda.gov/scripts/cdrh/cfdocs/cfcfr/cfrsearch.cfm?fr=314.80. Accessed June 5, 2014.

24. FiercePharma. Top 10 Generics Makers by 2012 Revenue. www.fiercepharma.com/special-reports/top-10-generics-makers-2012-revenue. Accessed June 5, 2014.

25. Academy of Managed Care Pharmacy. Guide to Pharmaceutical Payment Methods, 2009. *Journal of managed care pharmacy : JMCP.* 2009;15(6 Suppl A):S3.

26. King G, Donahoe G. Estimates of Medical Device Spending in the United States. AdvaMed; 2011.

27. Medical Product Outsourcing. The Medical Device Top 30—Your Online Source for Medical Device Product Information. www.mpo-mag.com/heaps/view/551/1/. Accessed June 5, 2014.

28. Maisel WH. Medical Device Regulation: An Introduction for the Practicing Physician. *Annals of Internal Medicine.* 2004;140(4):296.

29. Zuckerman DM, Brown P, et al. Medical Device Recalls and the FDA Approval Process. *Archives of Internal Medicine.* 2011;171(11):1006.

30. PricewaterhouseCoopers. Medical Technology Innovation Scorecard: The Race for Global Leadership. pwchealth.com/cgi-local/hregister.cgi?link=reg/innovation-scorecard.pdf. Accessed June 2, 2014.

31. U.S. Food and Drug Administration. Devices Approved in 2013. www.fda.gov/MedicalDevices/ProductsandMedicalProcedures/DeviceApprovalsandClearances/PMAApprovals/ucm344734.htm. Accessed June 4, 2014.

32. Maisel WH. Medical Device Regulation: An Introduction for the Practicing Physician. *Annals of Internal Medicine.* 2004;140(4):296.

33. Burton T. Recalls of Defective Medical Devices Nearly Doubled in Decade, FDA Says. *Wall Street Journal.* March 21, 2014.

34. Food and Drug Administration. Medical Device Recall Report. www.fda.gov/ downloads/AboutFDA/CentersOffices/OfficeofMedicalProductsandTobacco/CDRH/ CDRHTransparency/UCM388442.pdf. Accessed June 28, 2014.

35. Internal Revenue Service. Medical Device Excise Tax: Frequently Asked Questions. www.irs. gov/uac/Medical-Device-Excise-Tax:-Frequently-Asked-Questions. Accessed June 4, 2014.

36. Stewart-Williams S, Podd J. The Placebo Effect: Dissolving the Expectancy Versus Conditioning Debate. *Psychological bulletin.* 2004;130(2):324.

37. Melander H, Salmonson T, et al. A Regulatory Apologia—a Review of Placebo-Controlled Studies in Regulatory Submissions of New-Generation Antidepressants. *European Neuropsychopharmacology.* 2008;18(9):623.

38. Silberman S. Placebos Are Getting More Effective. Drugmakers Are Desperate to Know Why. *Wired Magazine.* 2009.

39. Ioannidis JPA. Contradicted and Initially Stronger Effects in Highly Cited Clinical Research. *JAMA: The Journal of the American Medical Association.* 2005;294(2):218.

40. Ioannidis JPA. Why Most Published Research Findings Are False. *PLoS medicine.* 2005;2(8):e124.

41. Emerson GB, Warme WJ, et al. Testing for the Presence of Positive-Outcome Bias in Peer Review: A Randomized Controlled Trial. *Archives of Internal Medicine.* 2010;170(21):1934.

42. Dwan K, Altman DG, et al. Systematic Review of the Empirical Evidence of Study Publication Bias and Outcome Reporting Bias. *PLoS One.* 2008;3(8):e3081.

43. Lexchin J, Bero LA, et al. Pharmaceutical Industry Sponsorship and Research Outcome and Quality: Systematic Review. *BMJ.* 2003;326(7400):1167.

44. Couzin J, Unger K. Cleaning up the Paper Trail. *Science.* 2006;312(5770):38.

45. Bachmann LM, Kolb E, et al. Accuracy of Ottawa Ankle Rules to Exclude Fractures of the Ankle and Mid-Foot: Systematic Review. *BMJ.* 2003;326(7386):417.

46. Graham ID, Stiell IG, et al. Awareness and Use of the Ottawa Ankle and Knee Rules in 5 Countries: Can Publication Alone Be Enough to Change Practice? *Annals of Emergency Medicine.* 2001;37(3):259.

47. McGlynn EA, Asch SM, et al. The Quality of Health Care Delivered to Adults in the United States. *New England Journal of Medicine.* 2003;348(26):2635.

48. Gardner B. The Crisis in Evidence-Based Medicine. *The Incidental Economist*; 2014.

49. American College of O-G. Practice Bulletin No. 122: Breast Cancer Screening. *Obstetrics and gynecology.* 2011;118(2 Pt 1):372.

50. U. S. Preventive Services Task Force. Screening for Breast Cancer: Task Force Recommendation Statement. *Annals of Internal Medicine.* 2009;151(10):716.

51. DiMasi JA, Grabowski HG. The Cost of Biopharmaceutical R&D: Is Biotech Different? *Managerial and Decision Economics.* 2007;28(45):469.

52. American Cancer Society. Clinical Trials: What You Need to Know. www. cancer.org/Treatment/TreatmentsandSideEffects/ClinicalTrials/ WhatYouNeedtoKnowaboutClinicalTrials/index.htm. Accessed June 2, 2014.

53. Gottlieb S. The FDA Is Evading the Law. *Wall Street Journal.* Dec 23, 2010.

54. Pollack A. Medical Treatment, out of Reach. *New York Times.* Feb 9, 2011.

55. Angell M. The Epidemic of Mental Illness: Why? *The New York Review of Books.* Jun 23, 2011.

56. Radley DC, Finkelstein SN, et al. Off-Label Prescribing among Office-Based Physicians. *Archives of Internal Medicine.* 2006;166(9):1021.

57. The Food and Drug Administration. Human Drugs Program. www.fda.gov/downloads/ AboutFDA/ReportsManualsForms/Reports/BudgetReports/UCM298355.pdf. Accessed June 5, 2014.

58. UpToDate. Rosuvastatin: Drug Information. www.uptodate.com/contents/rosuvastatin-drug-information. Accessed June 28, 2014.

59. Herper M. The World's Most Expensive Drugs. www.forbes.com/2010/02/19/expensive-drugs-cost-business-healthcare-rare-diseases.html. Accessed May 12, 2014.

60. Consumer Reports. Generic Drug Prices | How Drug Costs Compare. www.consumerreports.org/cro/magazine/2013/05/same-generic-drug-many-prices/index.htm. Accessed June 5, 2014.

61. Pharmaceutical Price Controls in OECD Countries. Implications for U.S. Consumers, Pricing, Research and Development, and Innovation. Vol 2011: International Trade Administration. US Department of Commerce. 2004.

62. Businessweek B. Merck & Co. Inc. (Mrk:New York): Financial Statements—Businessweek. investing.businessweek.com/research/stocks/financials/financials.asp?ticker=MRK. Accessed June 5, 2014.

63. Patent Full-Text Databases. Vol 2011: US Patent and Trademark Office; 2010.

64. Merck Announces Full-Year and Fourth-Quarter 2012 Financial Results | Merck Newsroom Home. www.mercknewsroom.com/press-release/corporate-news/merck-announces-full-year-and-fourth-quarter-2012-financial-results. Accessed June 5, 2014.

65. Merck Worldwide. Merck U.S. Prescription Products. www.merck.com/product/prescription-products/home.html. Accessed June 4, 2014.

66. Pharmaceutical Research and Manufacturers of America. Chart Pack: Biopharmaceuticals in Perspective. www.phrma.org/sites/default/files/pdf/CHART%20PACK_online%20version_13APR04_forweb.pdf. Accessed June 5, 2014.

67. Paul SM, Mytelka DS, et al. How to Improve R&D Productivity: The Pharmaceutical Industry's Grand Challenge. *Nature Reviews Drug Discovery.* 2010;9(3):203.

68. Persuading the Prescribers: Pharmaceutical Industry Marketing and Its Influence on Physicians and Patients—Pew Charitable Trusts. www.pewhealth.org/other-resource/persuading-the-prescribers-pharmaceutical-industry-marketing-and-its-influence-on-physicians-and-patients-85899439814. Accessed June 5, 2014.

69. AdvaMed. Comparison Chart: Advamed Code (2005), Revised Advamed Code (Eff. 7/1/2009) and Revised Phrmacode (Eff. 1/1/2009). www.advamed.org/res.download/138. Accessed June 5, 2014.

70. Friedman Y. Location of Pharmaceutical Innovation: 2000-2009. *Nature Reviews Drug Discovery.* 2010;9(11):835.

71. Rockoff J. Drug Reps Soften Their Sales Pitches. *Wall Street Journal.* Jan 10, 2012.

72. Campbell EG, Gruen RL, et al. A National Survey of Physician-Industry Relationships. *New England Journal of Medicine.* 2007;356(17):1742.

73. Healy W, Peterson R. Department of Justice Investigation of Orthopaedic Industry. *The Journal of Bone and Joint Surgery (American).* 2009;91(7):1791.

74. Centers for Medicare & Medicaid Services. Open Payments. www.cms.gov/Regulations-and-Guidance/Legislation/National-Physician-Payment-Transparency-Program/index.html. Accessed June 4, 2014.

75. FDA. Fast Track, Breakthrough Therapy, Accelerated Approval and Priority Review. www.fda.gov/forconsumers/byaudience/forpatientadvocates/speedingaccesstoimportantnewtherapies/ucm128291.htm. Accessed June 5, 2014.

Chapter 5
Policy and Reform

Disclaimer
This chapter is out of date.
It went out of date the second we sent it to the printer.

New research gets published every day, numbers get updated, debates switch focus. No matter how hard we have tried to include the latest numbers and evidence, no matter how hard we've tried to focus on what's happening as a *trend* rather than what's happening *now*, things will have changed by the time you read this. But the ground shifting beneath our feet tells us a few things.

▸ What's "obvious" may not be right (or may not work).
▸ What's right today might not be right tomorrow.
▸ We're all just going with our best guess.
▸ Don't get too bogged down in the moment—think of the past (has something similar happened before?) and the future (will the doomsayers look silly in retrospect?).
▸ Never be too sure of yourself (i.e., the data is ever-changing, almost every issue has a lot of nuance you might be missing, and the other side likely has good points).

This chapter focuses on the Affordable Care Act, but you should be thinking about health policy and reform more generally. Regardless of the ACA's specifics, reform is ongoing.

Health Policy

Public policy generally refers not just to laws but to the entire infrastructure of regulations, budgets, and planning priorities related to the implementation of a law. Health policy, then, is set at every level of government and can encompass everything from Medicare reimbursement rates to vaccine campaigns to NIH research funding to drug regulations to smoking bans. At its most basic, health policy seeks to design the financing and delivery of health care; beyond that, policy is created for a myriad of issues that affect public health.

With such a range of issues, you can imagine that many organizations are involved in creating and enforcing health policy. Some regulatory bodies create rules that have binding force—either in the court system or in licensing—while some make recommendations, and others lobby the political system.

Major Health Policy and Regulatory Bodies

GOVERNMENTAL

Department of Health & Human Services (HHS): This federal agency deals with almost all aspects of health in the U.S. The HHS Secretary sits in the Cabinet. Divisions include those listed below, along with non-health programs, like Head Start and Faith-Based and Neighborhood Partnerships. The HHS budget for 2014 was $950 billion (about $300 billion *more* than the Department of Defense, to give you a comparison),[1] which accounts for about one-quarter of the total federal budget.

Centers for Medicare & Medicaid Services (CMS): A division of HHS, CMS oversees, obviously, both Medicare and Medicaid, along with the State Children's Health Insurance Program (CHIP). It also administers the Health Insurance Portability and Accountability Act (HIPAA) as well as a number of quality standards in health care. Medicare is the nation's largest insurer, and many health care providers and facilities would have trouble getting enough patients to do business if they didn't accept Medicare. As such, Medicare has a lot of leverage over health care facilities and largely determines how the health care system is administered and financed.

Food and Drug Administration (FDA): A division of HHS, it oversees the safety of food products, pharmaceuticals, biologics, medical devices, and veterinary products. See Chapter 4 for more information.

National Institutes of Health (NIH): The NIH is the main government institution responsible for biomedical and health research; it's a major source of funding for medical research in the U.S. The NIH awards grants to medical researchers across the country, as well as employing and funding its own research staff. It maintains a number of centers and institutes, including the National Institute of Mental Health and the National Cancer Institute.

Centers for Disease Control and Prevention (CDC): The CDC is the primary government agency for public health and epidemiology. For example, the CDC is responsible for tracking and coordinating the national response to the spread of diseases such as influenza.

Agency for Healthcare Research and Quality (AHRQ): The AHRQ is the primary government agency for health systems and outcomes research. Studies focus on cost, access, and quality of U.S. health care. The AHRQ is a major resource for cataloguing clinical practice guidelines, as well.[2]

Surgeon General: The Surgeon General is the federal government's spokesperson to the nation on matters of health. He or she often spearheads large public health campaigns, such as encouraging Americans to quit smoking. The Surgeon General represents the U.S. government in a number of committees and private organizations and is the head of the Public Health Service Commissioned Corps.

Local Departments of Public Health (DPH): Not all health policy decisions are made at the federal level. Many are either decided or administered on the state or local level. The DPH is like HHS on the local level.

NONGOVERNMENTAL

Institute of Medicine (IOM): The IOM is a branch of the National Academy of Sciences. It's an independent, not-for-profit organization comprising academics and other health care experts that produces reports on topics relevant to the nation's health, such as childhood obesity and medical errors. Reports are commissioned and funded by a variety of sources, including the federal government and private organizations.

The Joint Commission (TJC): TJC is a nongovernmental, not-for-profit organization that accredits hospitals and other health care facilities in the U.S. Accreditation is dependent on adherence to a broad set of standards that cover everything from physician credentialing to placement of bathrooms. Although hospitals aren't required to be accredited by TJC, many government and private insurance programs will not reimburse non-accredited hospitals. Hospitals are examined by TJC for reaccreditation at least once every three years.[3]

American Medical Association (AMA): Established in 1847, the AMA is the largest and most powerful professional organization of U.S. physicians and medical students. While fewer than 20% of physicians today belong to the organization, most physicians are represented in the AMA by their respective specialty societies. Thus, it remains an influential force in both policy and politics. There are dozens of other professional organizations for all types of health care professionals.

Policy Research

Health policy impacts the lives of millions of people, so it's not surprising that a growing number of researchers are putting health systems "under the microscope" to see what works and what doesn't. Here are two examples of contemporary research with major policy implications.

OREGON MEDICAID EXPERIMENT

In 2008, Oregon had the funds to increase Medicaid enrollment by 10,000—but the state received 90,000 applications.[4] They decided to assign enrollment by lottery, randomizing who got insurance. That randomization meant that researchers had a pool of data to examine how insurance affects both health outcomes and utilization. In 2013, some of this research was published with the conclusions that "Medicaid coverage increased overall health care utilization, improved self-reported health, and reduced financial strain." Medicaid coverage did increase the diagnosis of depression as well as perceived mental health status. It did not, however, improve objective measurements of hypertension, high cholesterol, or diabetes, although it did increase medication usage for these conditions.[5] Later in 2013, further data from the Oregon Medicaid experiment was published, indicating that Medicaid coverage may increase rather than decrease emergency department (ED) visits.[6]

Critics of public health insurance—such as Avik Roy in *Forbes*—claim that these studies disprove the popular arguments in favor of expanding insurance coverage, (i.e., that insurance improves health status and reduces ED utilization and thus brings down overall health costs in the long run), and therefore that we should not be putting more patients into a "broken system."[7] Supporters of expanding Medicaid and other insurance coverage counter that the poor tend to have worse health, that the study was underpowered (i.e., the problem was with the statistics),[8] and that the ED usage rates might call for a concomitant "culture change" along with insurance coverage.[9]

GEOGRAPHIC VARIATION IN MEDICARE SPENDING

Since 1996, the Dartmouth Atlas has been cataloguing regional differences in Medicare spending. As it turns out, there are quite wide geographic variations—also known as unwarranted variations—in per-person spending even though Medicare has nearly identical pricing everywhere (unlike the private market). These differences in spending are diminished but not eliminated when one accounts for patient demographics such as age, sex, income, race— or health status.[10] Thus, higher spending regions provide more care but do not have better health outcomes. Many conclusions have been drawn from this information, i.e., that more care is not necessarily better care, and that clinical decisions may be influenced by forces outside of evidence or best practice guidelines. Such conclusions have made big press, including a high profile article by Atul Gawande comparing divergent spending in McAllen ($14,496 per beneficiary in 2006) and El Paso ($7,504 per beneficiary), two Texas towns with similar demographics and nearly identical health outcomes.[11]

In July 2013, the Institute of Medicine released a report, mandated by the ACA, looking at the same data as the Dartmouth Atlas. They agreed with the Dartmouth researchers that geographic variations are real, that they do not disappear when accounting for demographics, and that they are not explained by differences in health outcomes. Regions at the 90th percentile spend 42% more than regions at the 10th percentile, and differences in spending can mostly be attributed to acute and post-acute care (such as nursing homes or rehab centers). However, the IOM report notes that these differences persist no matter how small the geographic area is defined—concluding that differences come from institutions, not regions, and thus recommending against lowering Medicare reimbursement rates in high spending regions. The IOM report did recommend testing payment reform models and making data more available for further research.[12]

Elliott Fisher, one of the Dartmouth researchers, counters the IOM report, however, by emphasizing that many actions affecting population health occur on the regional or local level. He and other researchers still recommend regional policy efforts.[13]

Politics and Lobbying

Lobbying is a practice by which businesses, organizations, advocacy groups, and individuals try to inform and persuade the executive and legislative branches of federal, state, and local governments to vote or act in ways that promote or protect certain interests. Lobbyists may influence legislative and administrative bodies by sponsoring information sessions, helping to draft legislation, influencing the rules and regulations related to legislation, and contributing to political campaigns.

Health-related lobbying accounts for more spending than almost any other industry sector, outpacing even defense and energy lobbying.[14] As you can see below, some pretty large amounts of money get thrown around.

Lobbying Money (2013)		
Sector[15]	**Total Contributions**	**Top Three Contributors**
Pharmaceuticals and Health Products	$226 million	Pharmaceutical Research and Manufacturers of America: $17.8M Eli Lilly and Company: $9.8M Amgen, Inc.: $9.1M
Insurance	$153M	Blue Cross/Blue Shield: $12.9M America's Health Insurance Plans: $10.4M Prudential Financial: $7.4M
Hospitals and Nursing Homes	$91M	American Hospital Association: $19.1M Select Medical: $3.3M Federation of American Hospitals: $3.1M
Health Professionals	$84.5M	American Medical Association: $18.1M American College of Radiology: $3.8M American Dental Association: $2.8M
Health Services/HMOs	$68.9M	Blue Cross/Blue Shield: $5.6M Fresenius Medical Care: $4.7M Partnership for Quality Home Healthcare: $2.9M

Critics of such contributions suggest that they fuel ideological biases and conflicts of interest. However, just as with the physician–industry relationship, counterarguments may be made that these relationships play an important role in helping the system function.

Health Care Reform

National Reform Efforts

Health insurance legislation has a long, convoluted history in the U.S. We will give the most bare bones history of health care reform here, organized by what happened during presidential tenures. The U.S. health system has been haphazardly built through continual legislation, and interest groups (including physicians, insurance companies, businesses, and unions) have consistently opposed reforms. Think of a house that keeps getting new rooms and additions done by different architects and builders. It's a fascinating history, and, if you are interested in politics or history, we highly recommend reading Paul Starr (see Suggested Reading).

Late 1800s: Some European countries began enacting health insurance, either for the entire population or for subsets, such as workers.

Progressive Era (1910s–1920s): An advocacy group proposed legislation covering workers and their families for hospital and physician services, as well as for funeral benefits. However, diverse groups including physicians, private insurance companies, and labor unions opposed it, and it ultimately failed.

Franklin Roosevelt (1930s–1940s): Roosevelt passed the **Social Security Act in 1935,** which provided "old age insurance" (we call this social security), but he chose not to include health insurance as part of the Act because of how controversial it was.

Truman (1940s–1950s): Truman supported national, universal health insurance coverage in the late 1940s, but Congress consistently opposed it. During this time, our system of **employer-sponsored insurance (ESI,** see Chapter 2) developed, for two reasons. First, during World War II, the government limited wage increases but not benefits increases, meaning adding health insurance was a way to attract workers. Second, in 1954,

Congress decided not to tax ESI, making it cheaper for employers to provide health insurance than increase wages.

Kennedy & Johnson (1960s): Kennedy proposed Medicare but died before it could be passed; Johnson then pushed **Medicare and Medicaid** through Congress in 1965. Medicare, covering the elderly, was part of Social Security's "old age insurance." Medicaid, on the other hand, was insurance for welfare recipients administered jointly through federal and state governments, and which was optional for states to enact. This was the biggest piece of health legislation in U.S. history; in 1966, 19 million Americans were enrolled in Medicare and eight million in Medicaid. Notably, however, some states did not enact Medicaid right away. Arizona waited 17 years, leaving the care of indigent patients to the counties during that time.

Nixon (1960s–1970s): Nixon expanded Medicare eligibility to include those with end-stage renal disease (i.e., those who needed dialysis) and those with permanent disabilities who had been receiving Social Security for at least two years. This included two million more covered.

Carter (1970s): Carter wanted to pass comprehensive health insurance coverage, particularly because, by this time, many were critical of the "two tier system" set up by Medicare and Medicaid.[a] This was unsuccessful, but Medicare and Medicaid were moved into the same agency in 1977, when CMS was born.

Clinton (1990s): Clinton tried to push universal health coverage in 1993, but Congress rejected it. Two major reforms were enacted. First, the **Health Insurance Portability and Accountability Act (HIPAA),** which included various insurance reforms as well as broad health privacy laws. Second, the **State Children's Health Insurance Plan (CHIP),** which provided insurance to children whose families didn't qualify for Medicaid but couldn't afford private insurance.

The Second Bush (2000s): Bush created **Medicare Part D,** which extended pharmaceutical coverage to outpatient prescriptions. This benefit began in 2006.

---

a   As Paul Starr explains it, "The benefits that the elderly receive in the upper tier have been understood as an earned right, even though seniors have never paid enough in payroll taxes to earn their Insurance coverage (in fact, the first beneficiaries didn't pay anything). That moral claim has nonetheless given Medicare political security, making it unthinkable (at least until recently) to rescind the program, cap it, or cut it in a recession. In contrast, the recipients of Medicaid, like welfare, are not regarded as having earned any right, and that lack of a moral claim has made Medicaid politically Insecure and more vulnerable to cutbacks."

Obama (2000s–2010s): Obama passed the **Patient Protection and Affordable Care Act (also known as the ACA or ObamaCare),** the most significant piece of health legislation since Medicare. See most of the rest of this chapter for more information.[16]

State-Based Reforms

HAWAII

In 1974, Hawaii was the first state to enact near-universal health insurance coverage, with the Hawaii Prepaid Health Care Act (PHCA). The PHCA expanded employer-sponsored health insurance, mandating that businesses cover employees who work at least 20 hours per week.[17] (This type of "employer mandate" is also present in the ACA, although only for workers of 30+ hours per week.) Employers may self-insure or contract with private insurance companies, but either way the plans must be approved by the state. Employers further must pay at least 50% of the cost of premiums while the employees' share can't exceed 1.5% of wages. In 2012, 8% of Hawaiians were uninsured, a rate beat only by Massachusetts and Vermont.[18] (By comparison, the highest rate of uninsured was 24%, in Texas.[18]) Interestingly, research has shown that an usually high percentage of Hawaiians work less than 20 hours per week[19] compared to workers in other states, and the PHCA may play a role in this phenomenon.

MASSACHUSETTS

Massachusetts passed a comprehensive state health insurance reform law in 2006. Similar to the ACA (which was modeled on the Massachusetts law), it included an individual mandate to purchase health insurance, expansions of Medicaid and CHIP, the creation of health insurance marketplaces, subsidies for individuals below 300% of FPL (federal poverty level), reforms of the insurance markets, and new insurance requirements for employers, among other provisions.[20] The Massachusetts law has been in place for only a few years; however, intensive research has already been done to track the effects of the law on cost, access, and quality of health care within the state.[21] Here's a quick rundown.

The new law has dramatically increased health insurance coverage in the state. The percentage of non-elderly Massachusetts adults who are uninsured has dropped from 10.9% in 2006 to 6.3% in 2010,[22] but there is some question of how access to insurance has translated into access to care. Visits for specialist and preventive care have risen.[23] The increase in newly insured patients has put a strain on the primary care workforce, and wait times for new patients are longer in Massachusetts than in other states,[24] although more non-elderly adults in Massachusetts report having a "usual source of care" than in other states.[25] In the meantime, visits to the ED have also risen by up to 2.2%,[26] though they were expected to drop, while hospital admissions and readmissions have held steady.[27,28] There is also some evidence that preventable hospitalizations[29] have declined, and that racial and income disparities in access to procedures have improved.[28]

The follow-up question to this improved access is: Has it improved health status? Several researchers have conducted surveys of Massachusetts adults about health status, which have shown improvements in self-reported health[23] overall, along with other measures of physical and mental health and exercise.[30] A study in 2013 reported improved "general, physical, and mental health" in Massachusetts post-reform as compared to neighboring New England states.[31] Another study in 2014 found a decrease in mortality, both in total as well as in causes "amenable to health care," finding that one death was prevented for every 830 people who gained insurance.[32] (This was a big deal—especially in contrast to the Oregon Medicaid experiment, discussed in the "Health Policy" section of this chapter.)

Further, assessing the effect of reform on the costs of care is difficult because of the paucity of state-level cost data, the fact that costs for Medicaid expansion and other provisions of the law are shared between Massachusetts and the federal government, and the confounding effect of the financial crisis and recession that occurred at the same time reform was implemented. The weight of the evidence thus far has shown that care has become somewhat more affordable for patients.[23,33] The number of non-elderly adults who report not receiving needed medical care due to cost has decreased to 16.4%[25] (compared to 19.5% for the U.S. as a whole). The total share of debt and personal bankruptcies in Massachusetts has fallen as well.[34] At the state level, spending on health care has continued to rise, squeezing out government spending on education, infrastructure, and other service.[35] In response, the state government has passed a series of cost containment laws that are the most ambitious in the country, including statewide health care spending caps, alternative and quality-based payment systems, greater price transparency, broader roles for non-physician providers, and much more.[36] It remains to be seen if these measures will be effective in constraining health care costs.

Other Potential Reform Options

SINGLE PAYER

Proponents of single payer want a system in which all U.S. citizens are covered, with only one, government-run insurer. They claim that reducing the finances to a single payer would slash redundant—and quite expensive—administrative costs across the system. To point out that this could work, proponents suggest simply expanding Medicare to include everyone and eliminating private insurance; their slogan is "Medicare for all." This system would be similar to those of Canada, Japan, Singapore, and Taiwan. Note that single payer is not the same as "socialized medicine," because the delivery of care would still be privatized.

PUBLIC OPTION

Proponents of a public option support a government-run insurance system that may co-exist with private insurance, and citizens can choose between them. One way to achieve this would be to allow citizens of any age to enroll in Medicare. This system would be similar to those of Germany, France, and San Francisco (which has its own universal health coverage for city residents).

TAX BENEFITS AND INCENTIVES

Proponents of using tax benefits to expand coverage want to incentivize coverage without expanding the government's role. While there are many ways to change the tax code to incentivize coverage, one major suggestion is to make the tax benefits of employer-sponsored insurance (that is, the money spent on insurance one gets through work isn't taxed) available for anyone who purchases insurance. Other suggestions include tax write-offs for joining a gym or tax vouchers for those who truly cannot afford insurance on their own. This system is not similar to any other systems in industrialized nations.

PAYMENT REFORM

Proponents of the *many* payment reform options want to improve the system without having to overhaul it. The goal of payment reform is to reduce costs and incentivize better quality care. Some popular suggestions include Pay for Performance, Accountable Care Organizations, and bundled payments. We don't have the space to explore these here, but we suggest taking a look at the National Compendium on Payment Reform[37] to see all of the options out there, many of which are being tested as you read this.

The Affordable Care Act

History was made when Congress passed the Patient Protection and Affordable Care Act (ACA) and Health Care Education and Reconciliation Act (HERA), and President Barack Obama signed them into law on March 23, 2010. These laws represent the most sweeping changes to the government's role in the U.S. health care system since 1965.

To understand the basics of the ACA, let's look at a quick summary of how the law will affect major groups. After that, we'll use a Q&A format to answer some more in-depth questions about the law. Finally, we'll talk about the impact of the law, including financing and criticisms.

Quick Summary—How the ACA Affects Seven Major Groups

Federal Government

▶ The primary changes for the federal government center on Medicare, the establishment of a number of new organizations, and increased government spending on health care (with the hope of reaping savings on increased prevention and quality).

▶ The major Medicare changes are:

   ▶ Providing more preventive care without co-pays and deductibles

   ▶ Closing the Part D coverage gap (the "donut hole") through rebates and subsidies

   ▶ Freezing payments to some facilities and providers at 2010 levels for several years, while providing bonuses to primary care providers

   ▶ Testing delivery programs such as Accountable Care Organizations and medical homes

   ▶ Increasing the number of beneficiaries who pay higher premiums due to income

   ▶ Decreasing support for Medicare Advantage plans

▶ The federal government will make more payments for Medicaid, CHIP, and in subsidies to those with low incomes who purchase insurance through Health

(Continued) Federal Government

Insurance Marketplaces. These Marketplaces establish a portal for individuals and small employers to purchase insurance from qualified plans.

▸ Numerous new institutes and boards also have been created—too many to list in a summary—but they mainly focus on national quality and prevention strategies, greater coordination among institutions, comparative effectiveness research, and health workforce research. The federal government also will fund the newly created institutes, grants for states and businesses to develop innovative delivery systems, and tax breaks for small businesses that promote wellness.

State Governments

▸ The two major changes for state governments are:

  ▸ They may administer the Health Insurance Marketplaces; residents of states that opt out will use the federal government's Marketplace.

  ▸ States that accept federal money to expand eligibility for Medicaid and CHIP have additional requirements for how to administer these programs.

▸ States may decide whether or not to accept federal money in order to expand their Medicaid programs. If they do accept the money, then they must comply with the changes to Medicaid dictated by the ACA, including expanded eligibility* to include childless adults up to 138%[38] of the federal poverty level (FPL).

*For an explanation of Medicaid eligibility prior to 2014—and after 2014 in non-expanding states— see Chapter 2.

Insurers

▸ A number of restrictions are placed on insurers, most of which involve consumer protections:

  ▸ Insurers can no longer deny coverage for pre-existing conditions, end coverage when policyholders get sick, or charge higher premiums based on current or projected health status. Rating risk groups can now only utilize age, geographic location, family composition, and tobacco use.

  ▸ Insurers must keep their medical loss ratios (see Chapter 2) at 85% for large group and 80% for small group insurers, or else they must provide rebates to policyholders.

  ▸ Insurers must allow dependents up to age 26 to be covered under their parents' policies.

  ▸ Insurers may not place annual or lifetime limits on the amount they will pay out for policies.

  ▸ Insurers' plans must cover "essential health benefits."

▸ In addition, high-cost and consumer-driven insurance plans have new restrictions, most of which end tax breaks that individuals in these plans have enjoyed previously. Insurance companies get a deal, too: a huge increase in millions of new customers and government subsidies.

Employers

▸ The requirements on employers are different for large and small employers, so we'll look at those requirements separately. All employers must list the costs of health insurance for both the employer and employee on annual W-2 forms, and employers can offer rewards to their employees for participating in wellness programs and meeting health benchmarks.

▸ **Small employers (≤50 employees):** Receive tax credits if they offer insurance (only available for small employers with <25 employees), and they will be allowed to purchase insurance through the Small Business Health Options Program (SHOP), another Marketplace. They also will be able to apply for grants to establish employee wellness programs.

▸ **Large employers (51–200 employees):** Required to offer health insurance and, beginning in 2016, they will be penalized monetarily if they don't. Employers that do offer insurance may be penalized if premiums cost more than 8% of any full-time employee's income. (The point is to incentivize employers to provide affordable insurance.)

▸ **Very large employers (>200 employees):** Must automatically enroll employees in the company's health insurance plan, though employees may opt out.

Physicians

▸ Physicians will see their Medicare payments adjusted by 1% per the Value-Based Payment Modifier (see Chapter 2 for more information). Further, primary care physicians will see an increase in their payments, with a 10% bonus for services between 2011 and 2015, and an increase in Medicaid reimbursements to match those of Medicare in 2013 and 2014.

▸ The emphasis on new models of care such as Patient-Centered Medical Homes and Accountable Care Organizations (see Chapter 1) are likely to cause long-lasting changes in the way physicians work together and with other health care providers to deliver care.

▸ Finally, providers are likely to see more and better insured patients.

Hospitals

▸ Hospitals will be affected mostly by:

    ▸ Changes to the Medicare payment structure (including a pilot program for bundled payments),

    ▸ Decreased payments associated with hospital-acquired infections and readmissions (and thus a bigger push for quality),

    ▸ Loss of Disproportionate Share Hospital payments, and

    ▸ New requirements for not-for-profit hospitals (including quality measures).

Individuals

▸ The number one change is that it is easier for individuals to get insurance, and subsidies should make it cheaper or equivalent in cost for most people. This is accomplished by subsidies for the poor and near-poor, Medicaid expansion, mandates on employers to provide insurance, and regulation on the insurance industry. On the flip side, those who don't want insurance will be fined if they don't purchase it (with some exceptions).

▸ The law does a little bit of Robin Hood redistribution, too. There is a new tax on income above $200,000, and fewer out-of-pocket medical expenses can be deducted from taxes. On the other hand, Medicaid eligibility criteria widen (in cooperating states), and those who aren't eligible but make less than 400% of the federal poverty level can still get subsidies to purchase insurance through Marketplaces.

▸ For those who found insurance unaffordable or very difficult to qualify for based on their health status, things should get easier. Insurers can no longer discriminate based on pre-existing conditions or projected health status, and they can't limit the amount policies pay out in a year or in a lifetime. In addition, young adults will be able to stay on their parents' insurance until they're 26.

Businesses and Industry

▸ Health care reform places some haphazard regulations on business. This includes a 10% tax on indoor tanning and a tax on medical device and pharmaceutical companies. The FDA can now approve generic versions of biologic drugs. Chain restaurants must post caloric content on menus. And pharmaceutical companies that participate in Medicare will be required to offer discounts to beneficiaries who fall into the Part D coverage gap.

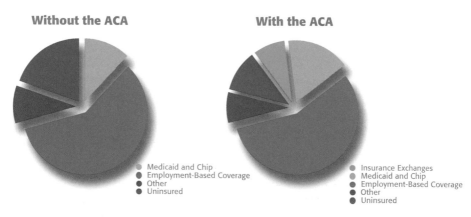

Projected Effects of the ACA on Health Insurance Coverage in 2024

Without the ACA

● Medicaid and Chip
● Employment-Based Coverage
● Other
● Uninsured

With the ACA

● Insurance Exchanges
● Medicaid and Chip
● Employment-Based Coverage
● Other
● Uninsured

Congressional Budget Office, "Insurance Coverage Provisions of the Affordable Care Act," Feb. 2014.
Note: Does not include those aged 65 or older.

Q&A About the Affordable Care Act

HOW WILL PEOPLE GET INSURANCE?

How to Get Coverage Beginning in 2014

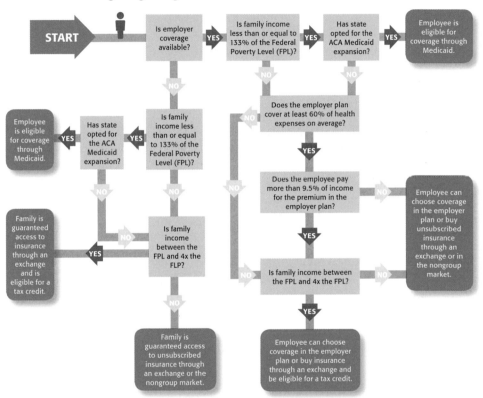

The Henry J. Kaiser Family Foundation, "Visualizing Health Policy: Health Coverage Under the Affordable Care Act," Dec. 2012. Used with permission.

WHO WILL STILL BE UNINSURED?

Some 30 million people will still be uninsured after the ACA is in full effect. This group is made up of:

▸ Undocumented immigrants
▸ Those who choose to pay the tax penalty rather than buy insurance
▸ Those who are eligible for Medicaid but choose not to enroll
▸ Individuals for whom insurance will cost more than 9.5%[39] of their

income (They may choose not to purchase it, and their fine is waived.)

▸ Those with income less than 138% of FPL (but who are not eligible for Medicaid at pre-ACA expansion levels) who live in states that chose not to expand Medicaid

WHAT IF I DON'T WANT TO PURCHASE HEALTH INSURANCE?

Beginning in 2014, all American citizens must be insured, and their insurance must provide "minimum essential coverage," also called "essential health benefits" (see later in the chapter). Those who do not have minimum essential coverage or qualify for an exemption will have to pay a tax (termed the "Individual Shared Responsibility Payment" by the IRS). The tax gets phased in, starting at $95 per adult/$47.50 per child in the household or 1% of income (whichever is greater) in the first year and topping out at $695 per adult/$347.50 per child in the household or 2.5% of income (again, whichever is greater) in 2016. Thereafter, it will increase with cost-of -living adjustments, though the penalty is capped at the amount of the average Bronze-level plan available in the Marketplaces.

Those who are uninsured for three consecutive months or less can apply for a "short coverage gap" exemption, but this can only be used once in a year. Otherwise, an individual must pay $\frac{1}{12}$th of the total penalty for each month he or she went uninsured in the prior year. The tax is either deducted from the person's tax return or put on a bill.[40]

Several groups are exempt from this "individual mandate" to obtain health insurance:

▸ People with financial hardship (e.g., any available plan costs more than 9.5% of your income)[41]

▸ People with religious objections (e.g., Christian Scientists)

▸ American Indians (who receive care through the federal Indian Health Service)

▸ Those who are uninsured for three months or less

▸ Those who are incarcerated (who receive care from the federal or state government)

WHAT IS A HEALTH INSURANCE MARKETPLACE?

A Marketplace[b] is a portal for purchasing individual health insurance. Think of it like using Travelocity or Priceline to purchase an airplane flight. The Marketplace offers certain private insurance plans under certain conditions, and you can choose the plan that works best for you.

Marketplaces offer plans in five levels:
- ▸ Platinum: premium accounts for 90% of the full actuarial value of the plan
- ▸ Gold: 80%
- ▸ Silver: 70%
- ▸ Bronze: 60%
- ▸ Catastrophic: This is a restricted level, as enrollees must be under the age of 30, and all other plans must exceed 8% of their income.[c]

That "full actuarial value of the plan" can be confusing. The Kaiser Family Foundation explains a Silver plan: "For a standard population, the plan will pay 70% of their health care expenses, while the enrollees themselves will pay 30% through some combination of deductibles, co-pays, and co-insurance. The higher the actuarial value, the less patient cost-sharing the plan will have, on average."[42] Thus, Platinum plans cost more in monthly premiums but cost less in co-pays and deductibles for services, and Bronze plans are the opposite.

In addition, every Marketplace does the following to make things easier on consumers:
- ▸ Requires plans to use "plain language" in written communication with the consumer
- ▸ Requires plans to explain what services have co-pays and deductibles
- ▸ Assigns a rating to each health plan based on relative quality and price
- ▸ Uses a uniform enrollment form and a standardized format to present benefit options
- ▸ Creates a calculator to determine the actual cost of a plan for each person, including tax credits, co-pays, and deductibles
- ▸ Provides a website where enrollees can compare information about each plan

b   This is the same thing as a Health Insurance Exchange, which you have also probably heard about.
c   Except for people with "substandard" plans cancelled at the end of 2013. They are allowed to purchase a catastrophic plan for 2014 only.

- ▸ Informs enrollees about their eligibility for Medicaid, CHIP, or other public programs and coordinates enrollment procedures with them
- ▸ Determines which individuals may be exempt from penalties if no affordable insurance plans are available through those individuals' employers or through the Marketplaces.

What subsidies are available to help people in need?

Folks who buy plans through the Marketplaces are eligible for subsidies if their income levels are between 138 and 400% of the federal poverty level and are based on the cost of the least expensive Silver plan available. The subsidies are provided as income tax credits or as a real-time monthly subsidy. These subsidies are based on the lowest cost Silver plan for your state's Marketplace, and they reduce premiums as indicated in the table below. Subsidies will be updated annually.

This table lists subsidies for a single, 40-year-old non-smoker who lives in an "average" state at different income levels.[43]

Income % of FPL	Cap on Premium Cost as % of Income	Annual Silver Plan Cost	Annual Government Tax Credit Subsidy	Annual Amount Paid for Premium
130%	2%	$3,240	$2,941	$299
150%	4%	$3,240	$2,551	$689
200%	6.3%	$3,240	$1,792	$1,448
250%	8.05%	$3,240	$928	$2,312
300–400%	9.5%	$3,240	$0	$3,240

Note: Tax credits also will be available for legal immigrants who aren't yet eligible for Medicaid because they have been citizens for fewer than five years.

HOW DID THE ACA AFFECT PREMIUM PRICES?

There isn't a simple—or a single—answer to this question.

First of all, premiums have long varied widely based on person as well as location, both before and after the Affordable Care Act. Second, answering the question involves comparing premiums across the Marketplaces, the private market, and employer-sponsored insurance, not all of which make data readily available to the public. Third, there isn't yet robust data, so most of what you read is anecdotal.

That being said, we can still give you some early numbers. In 2010, before the ACA took effect, Kaiser Family Foundation estimated the average U.S. premium price on the individual market to be $215/month (ranging from $136 in Alabama to $437 in Massachusetts).[106] The average employee contribution for employer-sponsored insurance was $93 monthly (ranging from $43 in Hawaii to $126 in Massachusetts).[44] Compare these numbers to the range in this graphic.

What Americans Pay for Health Insurance Under the ACA

The premium tax credit limits the amount an eligible enrollee would have to spend on a Silver plan, thereby reducing the variation in the cost of insurance.

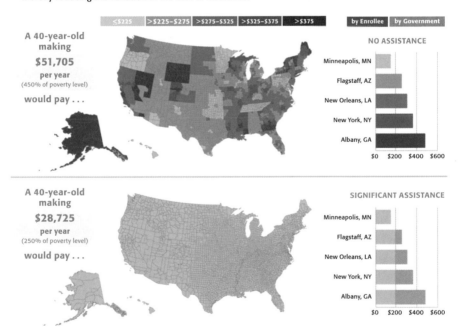

The premiums shown are for the second-lowest-cost Silver exchange plan available to a 40-year-old living in the county or region. Vermont and Massachusetts offer additional state-funded tax credits to eligible exchange enrollees (not shown).

The Henry J. Kaiser Family Foundation, "Visualizing Health Policy: What Americans Pay for Health Insurance Under the ACA," March 2014. Used with permission.

The bottom line is that some people are seeing their premiums change, and some aren't. This is one of those things that require patience for better data. In the meantime, some note that the focus shouldn't just be on premiums—as high deductibles represent a "hidden" cost. For instance, a plan with a $100/month premium may seem attractive, but it becomes less so when you realize it has a $5,000 deductible.

WHAT DO PLANS HAVE TO COVER NOW?

All plans must cover the following "essential health benefits": ambulatory, emergency, hospitalization, maternity and newborn, mental health and substance abuse, prescription drugs, laboratory, prevention and wellness, chronic disease management, rehabilitation and devices, and pediatric services. All plans must abide by general insurance guidelines concerning premium ratings (meaning insurers can't rate premiums on anything other than age, geographic location, family composition, and tobacco use).

WILL INSURERS STILL REJECT ME BECAUSE I HAVE A PRE-EXISTING CONDITION? WHAT PROTECTIONS ARE THERE FOR CONSUMERS NOW?

For many Americans, the new regulations on insurance aimed at protecting consumers will be the most noticeable changes of health care reform. The consumer protections on insurance include:

▸ Insurers can't deny coverage based on pre-existing conditions. (A pre-existing condition is a medical condition that began before insurance coverage began.[45])

▸ The waiting period for new insurance to take effect is capped at 90 days.

▸ Insurers may not cancel policies once policyholders get sick (aka "rescission").

▸ Insurers may not require co-pays or deductibles for preventive services (i.e., immunizations and screening for major diseases; must be rated Level A or B by the U.S. Preventive Services Task Force[46]).

▸ Deductibles may be no higher than $2,000 per individual and $4,000 per family, and total out-of-pocket costs are limited at $6,350 per individual and $12,700 per family.

▸ Insurers may not restrict how much they will reimburse claims either in a year or in a policyholder's entire life. In other words, insurers may not institute annual or lifetime limits.

▸ Insurers must maintain coverage for policyholders' adult, dependent children up to age 26.

In addition, insurance companies will be required to maintain a medical loss ratio of 85% for large group plans or 80% for small group and individual plans (or else provide rebates to policyholders), and insurance companies will be required to develop an appeals process and external review of health plan decisions. Thus policyholders may now appeal to their insurers when they think their plans are not up to snuff, and states must develop a board to review such plans.

WHY ARE SOME SAFETY-NET HOSPITALS WORRIED ABOUT THE ACA?

Hospitals that serve a large proportion of low-income patients (uninsured or covered by Medicaid) receive "disproportionate share hospitals" (DSH) payments. Providing care for this population leads to low or no reimbursement for the hospitals, so the federal government provides DSH to hospitals to help make up the difference. Medicaid DSH payments totaled $17.4 billion in 2011.[47,d]

Originally, since the ACA increases Medicaid eligibility and insurance enrollment, the law also decreased DSH payments (by complicated metrics which we won't go into here). However, Medicaid expansion is now optional, so DSH hospitals in states that are not expanding Medicaid are on the hook for the same number of uninsured and Medicaid patients yet no longer receiving the offsetting DSH payments.[48] Considering that safety-net hospitals already run slim margins, the financial pressure of DSH payment cuts may lead to layoffs, reduced services, or closures at affected hospitals in states that have chosen not to expand Medicaid.

The ACA only reduces DSH payments by $500 million at first, but the decline extends to $3 billion by 2020.[47] Affected hospitals lobbied against these cuts but were successful only in delaying them by one year, to begin in 2015.[49]

WHAT'S HAPPENING WITH HEALTH SAVINGS ACCOUNTS AND FLEXIBLE SPENDING ACCOUNTS?

Consumer-driven insurance includes such plans as flexible spending accounts (FSAs) and health saving accounts (HSAs). (See Chapter 2 for more information about these plans.) Tax-free contributions to FSAs are now capped at $2,500 each year, to be adjusted annually for inflation, and use of funds in FSAs is restricted to certain circumstances. In addition, FSAs

---

d   Medicare also makes DSH payments, which are calculated and distributed differently.

and HSAs can no longer be used for over-the-counter, nonprescription drugs (except insulin), and the tax penalty for using account funds for non-medical expenses increases from 10% to 20%.

I WORK FOR A SMALL BUSINESS—WILL MY EMPLOYER HAVE TO OFFER ME INSURANCE NOW?

It depends. Employer requirements for offering insurance depend on the size of the business and number of full-time employees. ("Full-time" is defined as working 30+ hours/week. Those working 29 hours or less are not required to be covered by ESI.)

If ≤50 full-time employees: Not required to provide employer-sponsored insurance (ESI). However, these employers are encouraged (with tax credits for businesses <25 employees) to provide ESI, either by purchasing it on the private market or through the Marketplaces. Employees not covered by ESI may purchase insurance through the Marketplaces and may be eligible for subsidies.

If 51–200 full-time employees: Must offer ESI.[e] Such businesses are penalized if (a) they don't offer ESI or (b) do offer ESI, but one or more employees are eligible to receive tax credits in the Marketplace (i.e., the ESI is unaffordable or the employees have very low incomes). The tax is $2,000 per full-time employee, minus the first 30 employees. Further, employers that offer coverage but have at least one full-time employee receiving a premium tax credit will pay the lesser of $3,000 per credit or $2,000 per full-time employee, again excluding the first 30.

If 200+ full-time employees: Automatic (opt-out) enrollment of all employees into ESI.

The ACA also incentivizes workplace wellness. Five-year grants are available to small employers who establish wellness programs, and employers are encouraged to offer rewards of 30% to 50% of the cost of coverage to employees for participating in and meeting certain health standards. (A few states may receive grants to try the same with private insurance, as with Marketplaces.)

---

e   The government issued two delays for the above businesses: Companies with 51–100 employees have until 2016 to provide ESI; and companies with 101–200 employees are only required to insure 70% of full-time employees.

CAN YOU GIVE ME A SUMMARY OF WHAT'S CHANGING WITH MEDICARE?

In terms of current Medicare beneficiaries, perhaps one of the biggest changes is that preventive services stopped requiring co-pays and deductibles as of January 2011. Such preventive services are rated by the USPSTF (U.S. Preventive Services Task Force) as having strong evidence of benefit; these include things like colorectal cancer screening, diet counseling, vaccinations, and depression screening.[50] The rationale (and this extends through health care reform in general, not just with Medicare) is to incentivize preventive care in the hope that this will make people healthier and reduce Medicare spending down the line by nipping costly chronic conditions in the bud.

Along the same lines (spending more now to improve the health of the population and hopefully decreasing long-term spending), Medicare has established or will establish several new programs. They are:

Accountable Care Organizations (ACOs): Medicare will allow ACOs to share in any savings they impart. See the next section for an explanation of what ACOs are.

Bundled Payments for Episodes of Care: This is a pilot program to give one lump sum for a course of treatment rather than the traditional fee-for-service payments. Four models are being tested in hospitals across the nation. For example, Medicare would pay $20,000 up front for the entire process of a hip replacement, rather than separate payments for the hospital, surgeon, anesthesiologist, hip implant, and rehab, as is currently the practice.

Independence at Home Demonstration Project: This pilot program pays physician and nurse practitioner teams to provide primary care services to underserved and chronically ill beneficiaries in their homes.[51] The program will last three years, and CMS will track the outcomes of affected patients.

Federal Coordinated Health Care Office: This office (created in 2010) identifies "dual eligibles"; that is, beneficiaries who are eligible for both Medicare and Medicaid. The office coordinates their care between the two programs. (Currently, everything is managed separately.)

Center for Medicare & Medicaid Innovation: This office, established in 2010, designs, models, and tests new delivery and payment systems for federal insurance programs with the goal of decreasing cost and increasing quality. Interestingly, it accepts suggestions from the public, which you can submit online.

CMS also will expand Medicare eligibility, though only in a very limited category. Medicare now will cover adults under age 65 who have developed health conditions following environmental hazard exposure in an emergency declaration area, though only for certain health conditions, and only for emergency declarations after June 17, 2009 (i.e., no Hurricane Katrina victims).

Further, in an effort to reduce fraud and abuse in Medicare (as well as in Medicaid and CHIP), CMS developed new levels of oversight in 2012. Providers, hospitals, and suppliers now will pay increased fees to fund these fraud prevention services. In addition, CMS can withhold payments to an organization if a fraud investigation against it is pending.[52]

WHAT IS AN ACCOUNTABLE CARE ORGANIZATION (ACO)?

An ACO is both a system of delivering care to patients and of receiving payment from insurers. Typically, providers are "enrolled" in the ACO, then patients who receive a plurality of their care are "attributed" to the provider and the ACO. As described in Chapter 1, this represents a "medical neighborhood" that includes primary care providers, specialty providers, and hospitals. The ACO coordinates patient care within an integrated infrastructure (e.g., same electronic health record, same billing system), and emphasizes primary care (e.g., easy access to a PCP who synthesizes all of your care within the network). The ACO is thus on the hook for patients (in terms of both cost and outcomes),[53] even if they see providers outside of the ACO network.

We won't go into the many different payment models here. The main point is that ACOs have an incentive to lower costs through the Medicare Shared Savings Program (MSSP).[54] Broadly, ACOs may receive bonus payments through the MSSP if they lower total costs (per attributed patient) below what they would be in a normal fee-for-service model. Pioneer ACOs—an early model including 23 ACOs[55] around the nation—may switch to a partial capitation model (thus taking on more risk).

Public health policy experts Drs. Mark McClellan and Elliot Fisher list the following defining principles of ACOs:[107]

▸ Provider-led organizations with a focus on primary care. The entire organization is accountable for quality and costs for all care that a population of patients receives.

▸ Payments are linked to quality, a move intended to reduce costs in the long term.

▸ The organization focuses on using performance measurements that are reliable, reproducible, and use data to improve over time. These performance measurements support improvements in care as well as savings based on those improvements.

▸ The goal of an ACO is to create "shared savings" for both the health care system and for the government. These savings will ideally accrue from improving the health of individuals and the population as a whole, and from decreased health care costs.

The idea of the ACO pre-dates the health care reform of 2010, but the ACA includes it as a function of Medicare and incentivizes it by allowing ACOs to share in any cost savings they produce. Some of the criteria ACOs must meet to share savings, though, are:

▸ Include at least 5,000 Medicare beneficiaries

▸ Agree to participate as an ACO for at least three years

▸ Maintain an overall management structure

▸ Develop processes to ensure the use of evidence-based medicine and quality measures

▸ Ensure patient-centeredness, as defined by clinician and patient surveys or by individualized care plans

WHAT'S HAPPENING WITH THE MEDICARE PART D "DONUT HOLE"?

Prior to 2014, there was a coverage gap for prescription drug costs between about $3,000[56] and $6,000[f] per year. Termed the "donut hole," this can get a little confusing. Patients' prescriptions were covered by insurance—meaning patients only had a co-pay—up until about $3,000, after which the patient had to pay for medications entirely out-of-pocket . . . until their costs reached $6,000, at which point prescription costs were covered by insurance again. As you can imagine, this has been a problem for many Medicare beneficiaries, not

---

f   Note that these dollar amounts were adjusted annually.

just those with low incomes but also those with chronic diseases that rack up prescription costs. The ACA aims to close the gap through several provisions:

▸ Pharmaceutical companies now provide a ~53% discount on brand-name, and federal subsidies provide a ~25% discount for generic prescriptions. (In 2013, this saved the average beneficiary "in the gap" $911.[57])

▸ Between 2010 and 2020, the federal government will roll out subsidies for brand-name prescriptions, with the goal of reducing patient out-of-pocket expenses on these drugs from 100% in 2010 to 25% in 2020.

WHAT CHANGES ARE BEING MADE TO MEDICARE SPENDING AND COST CONTROL?

Medicare costs have risen dramatically in the last two decades; the program already spends more than it takes in, and it's forecasted to run out of money in 2026.[58] (Though we should note that many such forecasts have come and gone through the years.) All of the expansions and added benefits listed above will cost money. As such, the ACA mandates some changes to how Medicare makes reimbursements to reduce spending.

The ACA also establishes the Medicare Independent Payment Advisory Board (IPAB). This board is tasked with recommending ways to reduce per capita Medicare spending if spending continues to grow past current targets. It will consist of 15 members appointed by the President and confirmed by the Senate. If Congress fails to enact the IPAB's recommendations, the HHS will do so independently, and Congress must act to override them. The IPAB has been controversial; it is opposed by the American Medical Association[59] and has been a target of Republican ire against the ACA. However, the IPAB can act only if spending growth outpaces targets—and, as of 2013, spending was below those targets. Thus, the IPAB may not end up being as important as projected.[60]

In the meantime, the ACA makes other changes to Medicare spending:
▸ **Value-Based Purchasing:** Adjusting payments to hospitals (and physicians) based on performance in certain quality measures. Further, the ACA mandates plans to implement value-based purchasing programs for nursing, home health, and outpatient surgical facilities. Implementation began in 2012. For more information, see Chapter 2.
▸ **Reducing payments to hospitals if they have excess readmissions.**

This is a measure to incentivize quality care both in the hospital and during follow-up after discharge. In addition, CMS counts readmissions to other hospitals, not just the original one. Implementation began in 2012. See Chapter 1 for more information.

▸ **Increasing Medicare payments for primary care services**—and for general surgeons operating in shortage areas—by 10%. This is both an incentive and a reward for primary care services, and the bonus payments last from 2011 to 2015. Granted, this isn't a measure to save on Medicare costs in particular, but it *is* part of the general thrust in the ACA to boost payments for preventive care in an effort to stem costs down the road.

▸ **Shifting more premium costs onto higher-income Medicare beneficiaries.** The income threshold for higher premiums in Part B will be frozen at 2010 levels until 2019, meaning it won't keep up with inflation, so more people will have higher premiums. The same provision will reduce the Part D subsidy (described earlier) for those with incomes above $85,000 per individual and $170,000 per couple.

WHAT CHANGES ARE HAPPENING TO MEDICAID AND CHIP AT THE FEDERAL LEVEL?

The general direction of the ACA changes for Medicaid and CHIP are to increase the number of people these programs cover, improve reimbursement, and test new care delivery models. Federal aspects of these changes are:

▸ For CHIP, to increase federal matching funds for states (increasing in 2015 by 23%–100%) and extend them until 2015).

▸ To encourage the expansion of Medicaid eligibility[g] in states by covering 100% of costs for these new enrollees from 2014 to 2016. The cost coverage will drop to 90% by 2020.

WHAT'S GOING ON WITH STATE MEDICAID EXPANSION?

Originally, the ACA mandated an eligibility expansion by offering a carrot or a stick: The federal government would initially cover all the costs of newly eligible enrollees, with a slight reduction over time—but, if states did not comply, then they would lose their federal Medicaid funding. However, in June 2012, the Supreme Court deemed this "stick" to be overly coercive to the states.

---

g   For information about eligibility when *not* expanded, see Chapter 2.

Now, states must comply with the new stipulations only if they accept the additional federal funding; otherwise, they are free to continue administering their Medicaid programs—and receiving the same federal funds—as before.

The main way the ACA expands access is by increasing eligibility for Medicaid (again, only in those states that voluntarily comply). New eligibility extends to uninsured individuals with incomes up to 138% of the federal poverty level.[38] This means that more low-income people will have access to Medicaid coverage. In addition, hospitals will be able to assume "presumptive eligibility" for patients they know to be eligible but are not already enrolled and bill Medicaid retroactively for their care.

Note, however, that increased federal matching funds will only cover these newly eligible enrollees; those who were previously eligible, even if they hadn't been signed up before, will be subject to the existing federal matching payments. In addition, the ACA requires states to maintain their current eligibility levels for children in Medicaid and CHIP until 2019, so states can't restrict eligibility for children's coverage in their efforts to stem spending.

As of June 2014, 27 states (including DC) are expanding Medicaid, four are undecided, and 20 are not expanding.[61] There is a strong "red state/blue state" correlation with the decision to expand, with the majority of non-expanding states being in the South and Midwest.

Where the States Stand on Medicaid Expansion

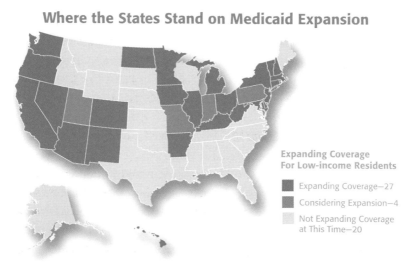

Expanding Coverage
For Low-income Residents

■ Expanding Coverage—27
■ Considering Expansion—4
□ Not Expanding Coverage
at This Time—20

The Henry J. Kaiser Family Foundation, "Status of State Action on the Medicaid Expansion Decision, 2014," June 2014. Used with permission. Note: Based on data as of June 10, 2014.

As health policy experts Drs. Benjamin Sommers and Arnold Epstein state in *The New England Journal of Medicine,* "The ACA requires the federal government to pay nearly the full cost of the Medicaid expansion (100% initially and 90% after 2019), and without this expansion millions of uninsured Americans would receive care from public clinics and hospitals that are subsidized by state dollars. So isn't the Medicaid expansion a winning proposition for states?"[108]

There have been several reasons cited by Medicaid expansion opponents:

▸ There is evidence that Medicaid provides poor access to the health care system compared to Medicare, and Medicaid coverage hasn't proven to improve health outcomes. (See the section on Oregon Medicaid Experiment.)

▸ There's no guarantee that the federal government will continue to pay 90% of costs for new Medicaid enrollees indefinitely—the states' share of costs may increase significantly with new budgets.[62]

▸ Medicaid already accounts for the largest share of state government spending at 25%[63] (ahead of K–12 education at 20%) and has been growing steadily. Adding more costs to this program (even if the federal government will pay for most of them) will put even more strain on already-tight state budgets.[64,65]

▸ To score political points.

WHAT ABOUT POOR PEOPLE IN STATES NOT EXPANDING MEDICAID?

The law does not provide for increased access to insurance for this population, and it is a serious concern. This situation came about because the law planned to expand coverage by giving Medicaid to everyone below 138% of FPL, and giving subsidies to those between 138%–400% of FPL. Thus, now that dozens of states are not expanding Medicaid, the law has no provisions to cover people who make less than 138% of FPL but were not *already* eligible for Medicaid. Keep in mind that Medicaid eligibility varies significantly state-to-state, and many states have strict eligibility rules. (In Alabama, for example, a single parent with one child would be eligible for Medicaid only if she made less than $236 a month,[66] and in 23 states, there is no Medicaid coverage for childless adults—even if they make zero income.[67]) Kaiser Family Foundation estimates that this leaves about five million poor adults in a "coverage gap."[68] (Twenty-two percent of this population will come from Texas alone.[69]) These people receive no additional help from the ACA to purchase insurance but are still subject to the tax penalty if they don't (although they may be exempt).

Interestingly, because of special circumstances of immigration law, new (legal) immigrants are the only members of this population who *can* get subsidies with incomes less than 138% of FPL.

WHAT ARE THE NEW MEDICAID PROGRAMS?

- **Medicaid Drug Rebate:** As of 2010, Medicaid receives a rebate of 23.1% of the cost of brand-name drugs and 13% of generics from drug manufacturers.
- **Money Follows the Person Demonstration Program:** This program, along with new initiatives for the Aging and Disability Resource Center, offers increased federal funds for Medicaid beneficiaries who move from long-term, live-in care facilities (e.g., nursing homes) to community-based locations (e.g., back home). The program has gone well since implementation; it now operates in 44 states and has covered 31,000 individuals.[70]
- **Extension of Medicaid Services to Homes and Community-Based Centers:** As of 2010, Medicaid covers the complete or partial cost of home- or community-based services, such as those by a home health aide or in a nursing home. Along the same lines, Medicaid will increase funding and services in home- and community-based long-term care, including for persons with disabilities.
- **Medicaid Payments Match Medicare:** Medicaid payments to primary care providers increase to equal the Medicare rates (which are typically 73% higher[71]) until the end of 2014.
- **Medical Home:** This program allows beneficiaries to designate specific primary care providers as "health homes" and offers 90% federal matching payments for two years for health home-related services. The Medicaid health home is based on the already existing concept of the Patient-Centered Medical Home (PCMH, see Chapter 1).

The above expansions and extensions of coverage will be costly. To help balance those costs, the ACA also mandates several decreases in Medicaid payments. In one major initiative, hospitals are no longer reimbursed for care related to health care-associated infections (HAIs, see Chapter 3). The ACA also will reduce states' Medicaid allotments for disproportionate share hospitals (those facilities that treat more Medicaid patients than average).

ARE THERE NEW INSURANCE TYPES?

There are three.

▸ **Indian Health Care Improvement Act:** This was a program that lapsed in 2001 and is now reinstated; it covers American Indians and Alaskan Natives and seeks to erase the health disparities in these populations versus the rest of the general population.

▸ **Consumer Operated and Oriented Plan (CO-OP):** Not-for-profit, member-run health insurance companies. Organizations can form their own plans and apply to be CO-OPs, but they must not be government-sponsored or already in existence as an insurer. They also must offer qualified health benefit plans and operate according to majority vote of members. Any profits must be funneled back to all members either through lowered costs or increased benefits. Twenty-three CO-OPs had been established by the end of 2013.[72]

▸ **Basic Health Plan:** This is an option for states to cover citizens earning under 200% of FPL but *not* eligible for Medicaid. The federal government will offer states 90% of what these citizens would have received in subsidies in the Marketplaces, and states can enroll them in Medicaid or in private plans. This option was delayed to 2015.

HOW DOES THE ACA ADDRESS RESEARCH?

Research is a major force not just in advancing care but also in developing efficient and valuable methods of delivering care. Thus, the ACA has established several new commissions to conduct research. Unfortunately, while it's (relatively) easy to establish a new organization, it's a whole other matter to fund and implement it, and many of the ACA's new commissions have not been funded.[h]

We should take note of one commission that did get funded: the Patient-Centered Outcomes Research Institute (PCORI). PCORI funds comparative effectiveness research, setting national research priorities and making sure the outcomes are useful to patients. PCORI awarded $316 million for 192 studies in its first three years.[73] PCORI is similar to England's National Institute for Health and Care Excellence (NICE), but, unlike NICE, PCORI is barred from taking cost into account in its recommendations.

---

h   Such as the National Health Care Workforce Commission and Research in Emergency and Trauma Medicine, for which Congress has not yet appropriated funds.

HOW DOES THE ACA ADDRESS THE UNDERSERVED?

One goal of the ACA is to improve primary care medicine, especially preventive services and care for underserved populations. The ACA introduced a number of programs on these fronts, including:

▸ **Strategies:** The development of the National Prevention Strategy and the National Quality Strategy, which are aimed at developing a cohesive plan for nationwide coordination of care and delivery.

▸ **Synchronizing Care for the Underserved:** Community-Based Collaborative Care Networks will encourage cooperation of health care providers to provide streamlined care for underserved populations.

▸ **Shifting Residencies to Primary Care:** Establish "Teaching Health Centers" by providing funding for primary care residencies in community-based, ambulatory health centers. The ACA also redistributes unfilled residency slots in specialty fields to outpatient, primary care settings. This doesn't increase the total number of residencies in the U.S., but it does prioritize primary care slots.

▸ **New Requirements for Not-For-Profit Hospitals:** Not-for-profit hospitals must conduct community needs assessments and develop plans for financial assistance to the needy. For those that don't meet these requirements, there will be a $50,000 annual tax.

▸ **More Money for Federally Qualified Health Centers** and the National Health Service Corps.

▸ **Workforce Shortages:** The Prevention and Public Health Fund aims to address primary care workforce shortages through training programs for low-income individuals wishing to enter the primary care workforce, as well as through wellness (focused on tobacco, obesity, etc.) and immunization campaigns.

▸ **340(b) Drug Discount Program:** This program provides savings of 20% to 50% on the cost of pharmaceuticals. Eligibility has been expanded to include safety-net hospitals.

DOES THE ACA ADDRESS DOCTORS' RELATIONSHIPS WITH INDUSTRY?

In Chapter 4, we discussed some of the issues involving financial relationships between industry, physicians, and researchers and how these can lead to conflicts of interest. The ACA seeks to shine a light on these financial relationships, without banning them, by requiring disclosure of financial relationships between health entities, including health care providers, hospitals, nursing homes, and manufacturers and distributors of medical goods. Any gift, sponsorship, or ongoing financial relationship must be reported to the federal government, which will in turn make the information available to the general public (see more on page 134).

What's the deal with provisions on tanning salons and restaurants? Beginning in 2014, food vendors and restaurants with more than 20 locations must post the caloric content of their food on all menus. They must also make information about saturated fats, sodium, and cholesterol available upon request. However, some businesses that sell food, such as movie theaters and bars, will be exempt. This provision has been delayed and final rules have not been published by HHS.

In addition, the law includes a 10% tax on indoor tanning services. You can think of this as a "sin tax," similar to the taxes on tobacco, which discourages use and offsets the costs that tanning might represent to the health care system long-term.

Financial Impact

CONGRESSIONAL BUDGET OFFICE ESTIMATES

Even now that the ACA has taken effect, it is important to keep in mind that almost all numbers about costs are just estimates. Here we will talk about estimates from the Congressional Budget Office (CBO), since it's a nonpartisan government agency that makes budgetary and economic projections. But different organizations make different projections. For instance, in 2010, the CBO projected that the ACA would decrease the deficit by $210 billion by 2021, while an article in *Health Affairs* projected that the deficit would increase by $500 million by 2019.[74] In truth, no one really knows what the financial consequences of the ACA will be.[i]

The CBO releases new predictions once it gets more information, so there have been a lot of numbers from them since 2010. Successive predictions have continually decreased how much the ACA is expected to cost. The most recent CBO projections suggest that the ACA will cost $1.4 trillion between 2014 and 2024[75] but will be "deficit neutral."

---

i   Which gives you a good reason to purchase the third edition of the *Handbook*.

The most recent CBO estimates as of this publication, from early 2014, include the following:[75]

▸ Access to insurance:
  ▸ Twenty-six million non-elderly adults will obtain health insurance due to the ACA by 2017.
  ▸ Thirty-one million non-elderly adults will remain uninsured. Forty-five percent will not purchase even though they could have access, 30% will be undocumented immigrants, 20% will be eligible for Medicaid but will not enroll, and 5% would have been eligible for Medicaid but live in a state that isn't expanding coverage.

▸ Effect on labor:
  ▸ Increased access to insurance will decrease the number of hours worked by the equivalent of two million jobs in 2017.[109]
    • Note that that is the "equivalent," because the number of jobs is not expected to change substantially, just the number of hours worked.

Budgetary Effects of the Insurance Coverage Provisions of the ACA, 2015-2024

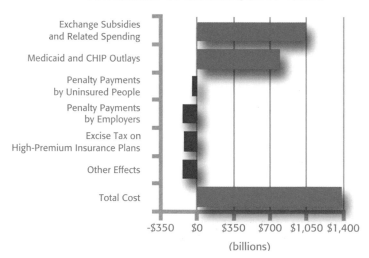

Congressional Budget Office, "Updated Estimates of the Effects of the Insurance Coverage Provisions of the Affordable Care Act," April 2014. Note: Positive numbers indicate an increase in the deficit; negative numbers indicate a decrease in the deficit. They exclude effects on the deficit of other provisions of the ACA that are not related to insurance coverage and federal administrative costs subject to appropriation. Effects on the deficit include the associated effects of changes in taxable compensation on revenues.

- Note, too, that this is not because businesses will demand less labor but rather because employees will choose to work less. As the CBO puts it, "workers will choose to supply less labor"[109] since they will have an easier time getting insurance without working full-time.

Of course, critics take issue with these estimates; any estimates you read will always have criticisms. But a criticism of particular note is that the CBO has a history of significantly underestimating the future costs of health care programs, including Medicare and Medicaid.[76]

NEW TAXES AND FEES

You may consider these Robin Hood measures, or you may consider them unfair taxation. Either way, they will help fund reform.

- ▸ Yearly fees on insurers. The fees total $8 billion in 2014 and increase to $14.3 billion by 2018.
- ▸ A temporary reinsurance program (lasting from 2014 to 2016), which accepts premiums from insurers in the individual market, as well as employers, and then provides payments to insurers who cover high-risk policyholders.
- ▸ An excise tax on insurers of employer-sponsored health plans with expenses that exceed $10,200 (single) or $27,500 (family). This is a way to garner revenue for reform while penalizing high-cost insurance, otherwise known as the "Cadillac tax."
- ▸ A 10% tax on indoor tanning services.
- ▸ Annual fees for pharmaceutical companies, totaling around $3 billion per year.[77]
- ▸ A 2.3% excise tax on the sale of any taxable medical device (e.g., pacemakers).
- ▸ The Medicare payroll tax rate increases by 0.9% (to 2.35% total) for all earnings over $200,000 for individual taxpayers and $250,000 for married couples. (There also will be a 3.8% assessment on unearned income for these taxpayers.)
- ▸ Individuals will be able to deduct unreimbursed medical expenses from their taxes only if these expenses are higher than 10% of income. The prior level was 7.5% of income. Individuals age 65 and older are allowed to keep this original level until 2016.

Impact of Health Care Reform

Issues with Implementation

THE FALL 2013 ROLLOUT BROUHAHA

Delayed Provisions

More than 20 of the law's provisions have been delayed. A few important ones are listed below. Note that more delays may be announced after publication!

- The "employer mandate," delayed by one year for large employers and by two years for mid-sized employers. Thus, employers will not be required to insure their employees in 2014. Why delay this part of the law? Because it also delays complaints from employers about cutting their workforce or cutting back on hours so they won't have to provide insurance for as many people.[78]
- The Small Business Health Options Program (SHOP[79]), delayed by one year. This is the employer version of the Marketplaces, which was set to launch in late 2013. Given the problems with the Marketplaces for individuals, HHS shifted workers from SHOP to the federal Marketplace for individuals in order to improve its functioning. The SHOP Marketplace is available to use through paper applications only.
- The deadline for purchasing insurance, delayed multiple times. For most people, this deadline was pushed back to mid-April 2014. For those who received cancellations in late 2013 of plans not meeting minimum essential coverage, though, the deadline is extended until 2016.
- Out-of-pocket maximums, delayed by one year for prescription drug plans not previously capping out-of-pocket costs. Such plans will not have to implement out-of-pocket maximums on prescriptions until 2015.[80]

The delays have been heavily criticized, not least from Speaker of the House Rep. John Boehner, who was quoted as saying, "What the hell is this, a joke?" in response to one of the delays. Republicans see it as a sign of bungled implementation of a bungled law. Further, there is a question of the legality of these delays, considering that the Executive Branch does not have limitless ability to enforce or not enforce statutes.[81]

Problems with the Marketplace Rollout

The Marketplaces were set to begin enrollment on October 1, 2013, with coverage beginning January 1, 2014. Some states created their own Marketplaces, while other states let the federal government establish their centrally run Marketplace (www.HealthCare.gov). When the Marketplace websites launched on October 1, it quickly became apparent that the federal Marketplace website had major problems. An estimated 8.1 million people visited the site,[82] with half a million attempting to create an account. The federal government faced heavy criticism for botching the rollout and turning away consumers, particularly with a deadline for when they must get insurance or face a penalty.

In response, the government extended the time for enrollment without a penalty[83] and worked to fix the website. Enrollment remained far below expected levels but picked up.

State-run Marketplaces generally did better than the federal Marketplace, with several seeing enrollment above expectations, including California, Colorado, Connecticut, and Rhode Island. On the other hand, some states had many more problems: Due to continued website glitches, Oregon had only enrolled 16% of expected consumers by January 1, 2014, and the website was still not operational.[84]

By April 2014, up to eight million people had enrolled in Marketplaces, 28% of the new enrollees being "young" (i.e., between the ages of 18–34).[85] The majority of these new consumers—60%—enrolled in Silver plans.[86] This meets the Administration's goals of seven million enrollees by the end of March and 25% young enrollees; however, certain aspects remain to be seen. First, there is no data on how many of the new enrollees were previously uninsured (which is relevant to the goal of decreasing the number of uninsured);[87] second, what the Marketplaces really need are healthy enrollees ("young" is just a proxy for "healthy"), and we don't know yet whether enrollees will be on average healthy enough to keep premiums low. Moreover, it appears that 10–20% of these folks weren't paying up—putting actual enrollment a little lower.[88,89] (Keep in mind these numbers are likely to change 20 times by the time you read this, so don't blame consumers too readily.)

Many have compared the Marketplace rollout with similar problems that Medicare Part D had during its launch under President George W. Bush in 2005. In that case, a botched launch had no long-term impact on the success of the program, and supporters claim that the Marketplaces will be the same.

ENROLLMENT BY THE DEADLINE

This is a tougher number to estimate than you might think, considering there is no registry or tracking of the insured. We do, however, have a few numbers for you. First, the Urban Institute estimates that the number of uninsured fell by 5.4 million from 2013 to March 2014.[90] That number takes into account all types of coverage, with the major two being Medicaid expansion and the Marketplaces. The uninsured rate has dropped further in states expanding Medicaid than in those that haven't.[90]

Second, a June 2014 Gallup poll found that "five percent of Americans report being newly insured in 2014. More than half of that group, or 2.8% of the total U.S. population, say they got their new insurance through the health exchanges that were open through mid-April."[110]

A few more numbers:
▸ Medicaid expansion (along with CHIP) is estimated to have covered about three million extra people, out of 11.7 million newly eligible.[91]
▸ The Marketplaces enrolled 7.1 million people by the deadline, just beating the CBO estimate of seven million from the prior year.[92] (The CBO predicts that Marketplace enrollment will

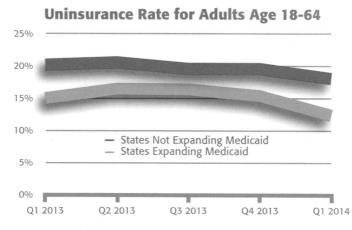

Uninsurance Rate for Adults Age 18-64

States Not Expanding Medicaid
States Expanding Medicaid

Long, et al., "Quick Take: Number of Uninsured Adults Falls by 5.4 Million since 2013," April 2014. Used with permission. Note: Medicaid expansion decisions as of April 1, 2014.

continue to rise until about 24–25 million in 2017.[93])
- ‣ Dependent coverage (which started in 2012) included three million adults under age 26.[94]

However, when talking about the numbers of enrollees, it's important to ask how many of these enrollees were previously uninsured. McKinsey, for instance, estimated in March 2014 (before the deadline) that only 14% of Marketplace enrollees had been previously uninsured.[95] Finding out all of the true—and relevant—numbers will take time.

Criticisms of the Affordable Care Act

We are not endorsing these positions, and there are counterpoints to all of them. This section simply gives a voice to the ACA's critics, in their own words, so you can see the range of opinion out there.

It will make health insurance more expensive: "The law forces insurers to charge the same rates to the healthy and the sick. It mandates that insurers cover services that the government deems 'essential,' such as drug-addiction therapy, that most people don't need. It forces young people to pay much more, so as to partially subsidize the elderly. There's no such thing as a free lunch. All these new rules [will] make health insurance more expensive."[96]

It will increase government debt: "The Patient Protection and Affordable Care Act is fiscally dangerous at a moment when the United States is already facing a sea of red ink. It creates a massive new entitlement at a time when the budget is already buckling under the weight of existing entitlements. At a minimum, it will add $1 trillion to government spending over the next decade. Assertions that these costs are paid for are based on omitted costs, budgetary gimmicks, shifted premiums from other entitlements, and unsustainable spending cuts and revenue increases."[97]

It narrows networks too much: "[T]he rules ObamaCare imposes to create a supposedly superior *insurance* product are resulting in an objectively inferior *medical* product. The new mandates and rules raise costs, so insurers must compensate by offering narrow and less costly networks of doctors, hospitals and other providers in their ObamaCare products. Insurers thus restrict care and patient choice of physicians in exchange for discounted reimbursement rates, much as Medicaid does . . . [e]verybody gets 'free' preventive checkups with no copays, but not treatment for a complex illness from specialists at an academic medical center."[98]

It leads to more government regulation and less free-market competition: "Americans want to have choice and control over their health care (including the doctors they want to see) and want those who provide health care services—insurers, hospitals, and other health care providers—to compete to provide them better care at lower prices . . . [ObamaCare] depends on a complex system of government mandates, inter-dependent regulations, and a highly involved, never-ending process of government decision-making that ultimately takes personal health care decisions out of the hands of American citizens."[99]

It is inefficient: "Obamacare was sold as a response to the alleged emergency presented by 40-odd million Americans' lacking insurance. That number was hotly disputed at the time, but even if we were to take it at face value, getting the figure down to 30 million at a cost of more than $1 trillion is hardly a bargain."[100]

These are mostly criticisms from the political right. But the ACA doesn't lack for critics on the left, too. . . .

It doesn't go far enough: "[The ACA's] approach to health care is fundamentally flawed. It is exceedingly complex. It perpetuates and entrenches the inefficient insurance model of payment for health care. It does nothing to address the rapacious pricing of pharmaceuticals. It ignores hospitals' 'medical arms race,' in which they expand facilities and services based not on community need, but on potential for profit. It still burdens doctors and hospitals with multiple payers, abstruse coding and insecurity about payment for delivered services. It is subject to state-by-state sabotage. At its most optimistic projection it leaves at least 25 million people [uninsured]."[101]

Challenges to the ACA

THE REPUBLICAN RESPONSE

Mostly, this response has consisted of numerous attempts at repeal. As of the end of 2013, the House voted 47 times to repeal the ACA, although none of these attempts got much traction in the Senate. One of the criticisms of the Republicans was that their position never offered an alternative to the ACA—until, in early 2014, Senate Republicans proposed a comprehensive reform plan to replace "ObamaCare."[102]

Here's the plan in a nutshell, and the corresponding aspects of the ACA.

Republican Replacement Plan	ACA
▸ Ends pre-existing exclusions for anyone who is continuously insured.[j]	▸ The ACA disallows any consideration of pre-existing conditions, regardless of prior coverage.
▸ Incentivizes insurance by the above—i.e., you should remain insured because, if you don't, your insurance will be much more expensive if you develop a condition and then want insurance.	▸ The ACA incentivizes coverage by imposing a tax penalty for anyone who wasn't insured in the past year.
▸ Makes insurance more affordable by offering subsidies up to 300% of FPL.	▸ The ACA makes insurance more affordable by expanding access to Medicaid up to 138% of FPL (in states that choose to do so), then offering subsidies between 138–400% of FPL.
▸ Pays for the above by restricting the tax-protected status of employer-sponsored insurance[k] (ESI, see Chapter 2), "cap[ping] the tax exclusion at 65% of the cost of an average health plan."[103]	▸ The ACA pays for the expansion in Medicaid and for subsidies through a myriad of changes, mostly taxes on industry and on expensive, "Cadillac" insurance plans. It lets ESI retain tax-free status.
▸ Allows states to auto-enroll residents into insurance plans if they are eligible for premium tax credits.	▸ No auto-enrollment.
▸ Restricts Medicaid eligibility.	▸ Expands Medicaid eligibility.

---

j   Note that, since 1996, HIPAA has done something similar, making pre-existing conditions much less of a concern if one has been continuously insured, as through an employer. As the AHRQ puts it, "Insurers can impose only a 12-month waiting period for any preexisting condition that has been diagnosed or treated within the preceding 6 months. As long as you have maintained continuous coverage without a break of more than 63 days, your prior health insurance coverage will be credited toward the preexisting condition exclusion period," meaning that for someone, say, switching jobs without any gap in insurance coverage, a pre-existing condition like diabetes is not a concern. That's *pre*-ACA.

k   To give a little background: Both pre- and post-ACA, any money put toward ESI is tax-free, making it cheaper. Economists have long argued against this practice, and the Republican plan seeks to end it, effectively leveling the playing field between those who get insurance through their jobs and those who get insurance on the private market.

COURT CHALLENGES

Scores of lawsuits have challenged health care reform—the first was filed just seven minutes after the ACA was signed into law—and the issue made its way to the Supreme Court. In March 2012, the Supreme Court heard arguments on four issues, and, in June 2012, the Court released the opinions. The two major decisions were:

1. The Court struck down the mandatory expansion of Medicaid. The Court decided that the ACA was overly coercive to states by threatening to take away *all* Medicaid funding if states did not expand eligibility. Thus, this part of the law was struck down, freeing states to choose whether or not to expand Medicaid eligibility. If they choose to and accept additional federal money, they must comply with the ACA rules about it. If they choose not to, they will still receive the same historical federal funding for the same Medicaid programs as before.

2. The Court upheld that individual mandate is allowed by the Constitution. The majority opinion held that the individual mandate is constitutional *if* defined as a tax penalty.

There have been a number of other unsuccessful challenges in the lower courts. In 2014, the biggest legal challenge involved technical language of the law. Cases in several states, including *Halbig v. Sebelius* in DC, contend that the law is written such that the government can offer subsidies through the Marketplaces only if those Marketplaces are run by the states. Considering that 34 states have federally run Marketplaces, covering 80% of the consumers receiving subsidies,[104] this presents a serious challenge to the viability of the law.

Another legal challenge doesn't involve the law as a whole but does threaten its required benefits—namely of contraception. *Sebelius v. Hobby Lobby* argues that, under religious freedom, employers should not have to contribute to insurance that provides contraception.

Public Opinion of the Affordable Care Act[1]

Public opinion on reform runs the gamut from people who think it fails because it doesn't establish single-payer nationalized health insurance to people who think it fails because it exists at all. As you can see, levels of support and opposition to the ACA have been neck-and-neck since the law was passed.

Three Years of Closely Divided Opinion on the ACA

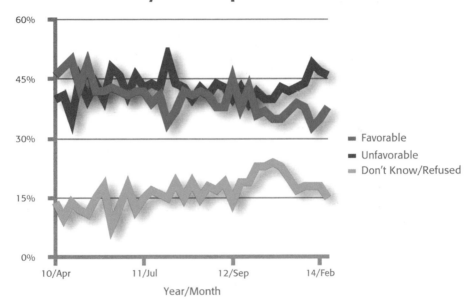

Hamel, Firth, and Brodie, "Kaiser Health Tracking Poll: March 2014," March 2014.
Used with permission.

On the other hand, if you break down the law to its elements, these are remarkably popular across party lines, and increasing in popularity over time.[105]

One of the main goals of the ACA was to help the uninsured, so it may come as a surprise that most uninsured Americans neither like nor understand the law. As of March 2014 (the deadline month for signing up) only 67% of the uninsured had even attempted to obtain coverage.[105] Some of that was ignorance of deadlines, but others intend to remain uninsured.

---

1   kff.org/health-reform/poll-finding/kaiser-health-tracking-poll-february-2014/

Percent "favorable" opinion of each provision	Total	Democrats	Independents	Republicans
Extension of Dependent Coverage	80	87	76	76
Closing Medicare "Donut Hole"	79	89	75	73
Subsidy Assistance	77	89	74	65
Eliminating Out-of-Pocket Costs For Preventive Services	77	81	76	75
Medicaid Expansion	74	89	69	62
Guaranteed Issue	70	74	70	69
Medical Loss Ratio	62	68	64	54
Increasing Medicare Payroll Tax on Those with Higher Incomes	56	77	54	33
Individual Mandate	35	56	31	16

So people aren't crazy about the ACA. Are they burned up about it? Do they want to get rid of it? Not really.

Not only that, but people are sick of hearing about it. Fifty-eight percent of Democrats—and 47% of Republicans!—say they are tired of the debate and want to focus on other issues.[105]

Share of Adults Age 18-64 with an Unfavorable View of the ACA

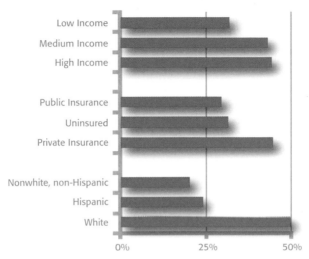

Adapted from: Holahan, et al., "Health Reform Monitoring Summary,"
Feb. 2014. Used with permission. Note: Low Income = Less than or equal to 138% of
FPL; Medium = 139–399% FPL; High = 400% FPL or more.

What Should be Done with the ACA?

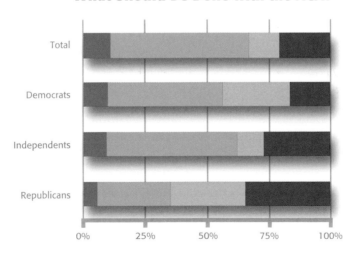

- ■ Keep the Law as it is
- ■ Keep the Law in Place and Work to Improve it
- ■ Repeal the Law and Replace it with a Republican-sponsored Alternative
- ■ Repeal the Law and Not Replace it

Hamel, Firth, and Brodie, "Kaiser Health Tracking Poll: March 2014,"
March 2014. Used with permission. Note: None of these/They should do
something else and Don't know/Refused answers not shown.

References

1.   The Associated Press. An Agency-by-Agency Guide to Obama's 2014 Budget. bigstory. ap.org/article/agency-agency-guide-obamas-2014-budget. Accessed July 15, 2014.

2.   Agency for Healthcare Research and Quality. National Guideline Clearinghouse. www. guideline.gov/. Accessed July 15, 2014.

3.   The Joint Commission. Joint Commission FAQ Page. www.jointcommission.org/about/ JointCommissionFaqs.aspx?CategoryId=10. Accessed July 15, 2014.

4.   The National Bureau of Economic Research. The Oregon Health Insurance Experiment— Study Information. www.nber.org/oregon/study_information.html. Accessed July 15, 2014.

5.   Baicker K, Taubman S, et al. The Oregon Experiment—Effects of Medicaid on Clinical Outcomes. *New England Journal of Medicine.* 2013;368:1713.

6.   Taubman S, Allen HL, et al. Medicaid Increases Emergency-Department Use: Evidence from Oregon's Health Insurance Experiment. *American Association for the Advancement of Science.* 2014-01-17;343(6168):263.

7.   Avik R. Oregon Study: Medicaid 'Had No Significant Effect' on Health Outcomes Vs. Being Uninsured. *Forbes* 2013.

8.   Carroll A, Frakt A. Oregon Medicaid—Power Problems Are Important. theincidentaleconomist.com/wordpress/oregon-medicaid-power-problems-are-important/. Accessed July 21, 2014.

9.   Frakt A. A Few Thoughts on the Latest Oregon Medicaid Results. theincidentaleconomist.com/ wordpress/a-few-thoughts-on-the-latest-oregon-medicaid-results/. Accessed July 21, 2014.

10.   The Dartmouth Atlas of Health Care. Understanding of the Efficiency and Effectiveness of the Health Care System. www.dartmouthatlas.org/. Accessed July 15, 2014.

11.   Gawande A. The Cost Conundrum. *The New Yorker.* June 1, 2009.

12.   Institute of Medicine of the National Academies. Variation in Health Care Spending: Target Decision Making, Not Geography. www.iom.edu/Reports/2013/Variation-in-Health-Care-Spending-Target-Decision-Making-Not-Geography.aspx. Accessed July 15, 2014.

13.   Fisher E, Skinner J. Making Sense of Geographic Variations in Health Care: The New IOM Report. *Health Affairs;* 2013.

14.   Center for Responsive Politics. Influence and Lobbying. www.opensecrets.org/industries/. Accessed July 12, 2014.

15.   OpenSecrets.org. Lobbying Spending Database Pharmaceuticals/Health Products. www. opensecrets.org/lobby/indusclient.php?id=H04&year=2013. Accessed July 21, 2014.

16.   Centers for Medicare & Medicaid Services. Tracing the History of CMS Programs: From President Theodore Roosevelt to President George W. Bush. www.cms.gov/About-CMS/ Agency-Information/History/Downloads/PresidentCMSMilestones.pdf. Accessed July 21, 2014.

17.   Library of Congress. State Legislation on Comprehensive Health Care Coverage: Hawaii. www.loc.gov/law/help/statehealthplans/hawaii.php. Accessed July 15, 2014.

18.   The Henry J. Kaiser Family Foundation. Health Insurance Coverage of the Total Population. kff.org/other/state-indicator/total-population/. Accessed July 8, 2014.

19.   Buchmueller T, DiNardo J, et al. The Effect of an Employer Health Insurance Mandate on Health Insurance Coverage and the Demand for Labor: Evidence from Hawaii. Institute for the Study of Labor; 2009.

20.   The 188th General Court of The Commonwealth of Massachusetts. An Act Providing Access to Affordable, Quality, Accountable Health Care. malegislature.gov/Laws/ SessionLaws/Acts/2006/Chapter58. Accessed July 21, 2014.

21.   Long SK, Stockley K, et al. National Reform: What Can We Learn from Evaluations of Massachusetts? www.shadac.org/files/shadac/publications/ MassachusettsNationalLessonsBrief.pdf. Accessed July 21, 2014.

22. The Henry J. Kaiser Family Foundation. Massachusetts Health Care Reform: Six Years Later. www.kaiserfamilyfoundation.files.wordpress.com/2013/01/8311.pdf. Accessed July 21, 2014.

23. Long SK, Stockley K, et al. Massachusetts Health Reforms: Uninsurance Remains Low, Self-Reported Health Status Improves as State Prepares to Tackle Costs. *Health Affairs.* 2012;31(2):444.

24. Rhodes KV, Kenney GM, et al. Primary Care Access for New Patients on the Eve of Health Care Reform. *JAMA Internal Medicine.* 2014/06/01 2014;174(6):861.

25. Blue Cross Massachusetts Foundation. 2012 Massachusetts Health Reform Survey. bluecrossmafoundation.org/publication/2012-massachusetts-health-reform-survey. Accessed July 21, 2014.

26. Smulowitz PB, O'Malley J, et al. Increased Use of the Emergency Department after Health Care Reform in Massachusetts. *Annals of Emergency Medicine.* 2014.

27. Hanchate AD, McCormick D, et al. Abstract 23: Impact of Massachusetts Health Reform on Hospitalizations, Length of Stay and Costs of Inpatient Care: Does Safety-Net Status Matter? *American Heart Association.* 2014.

28. Lasser KE, Hanchate AD, et al. The Effect of Massachusetts Health Reform on 30 Day Hospital Readmissions: Retrospective Analysis of Hospital Episode Statistics. *British Medical Journal.* 2014;348.

29. Kolstad JT, Kowalski AE. The Impact of Health Care Reform on Hospital and Preventive Care: Evidence from Massachusetts. The National Bureau of Economic Research; 2010.

30. Courtemanche CJ, Zapata D. Does Universal Coverage Improve Health? The Massachusetts Experience. www.nber.org/papers/w17893: National Bureau of Economics Research. Accessed July 21, 2014.

31. Van Der Wees PJ, Zaslavsky AM, et al. Improvements in Health Status after Massachusetts Health Care Reform. *Milbank Quarterly.* Dec 2013;91(4):663.

32. Sommers B, Long S, et al. Changes in Mortality after Massachusetts Health Care Reform: A Quasi-Experimental Study. *Annals of Internal Medicine.* 2014/05/06;160(9):585.

33. Himmelstein DU, Thorne D, et al. Medical Bankruptcy in Massachusetts: Has Health Reform Made a Difference? *The American Journal of Medicine.* 2011;124(3):224.

34. Mazumder B, Miller S. The Effects of the Massachusetts Health Reform on Financial Distress. Federal Reserve Bank of Chicago; 2014.

35. Health Policy Commission. 2013 Cost Trends Report. www.mass.gov/anf/docs/hpc/2013-cost-trends-report-final.pdf. Accessed July 21, 2014.

36. The Next Phase of Massachusetts Health Care Reform. www.mass.gov/governor/agenda/healthcare/cost-containment/health-care-cost-containment-legislative-summary.pdf. Accessed July 21, 2014.

37. Catalyst for Payment Reform. National Compendium on Payment Reform. compendium.catalyzepaymentreform.org/home. Accessed July 21, 2014.

38. State Health Access Data Assistance Center. ACA Note: When 133 Equals 138—FPL Calculations in the Affordable Care Act | State Health Access Data Assistance Center. www.shadac.org/blog/aca-note-when-133-equals-138-fpl-calculations-in-affordable-care-act. Accessed July 21, 2014.

39. The Henry J. Kaiser Family Foundation. What Americans Pay for Health Insurance under the ACA. www.kff.org/slideshow/what-americans-pay-for-health-insurance-under-the-aca-jama-march-19-2014/. Accessed July 21, 2014.

40. Internal Revenue Service. The Individual Shared Responsibility Provision. www.irs.gov/uac/Individual-Shared-Responsibility-Provision. Accessed July 21, 2014.

41. Appleby J. For 3 million, 'Affordable' Health Care Might Not Be. *USA Today.* Feb 8, 2014.

42. The Henry J. Kaiser Family Foundation. What the Actuarial Values in the Affordable Care Act Mean. kaiserfamilyfoundation.files.wordpress.com/2013/01/8177.pdf. Accessed July 21, 2014.

43. The Henry J. Kaiser Family Foundation. Subsidy Calculator. kff.org/interactive/subsidy-calculator/. Accessed July 21, 2014.

44. The Henry J. Kaiser Family Foundation. Average Single Premium per Enrolled Employee For Employer-Based Health Insurance. kff.org/other/state-indicator/single-coverage/. Accessed July 21, 2014.

45. The Henry J. Kaiser Family Foundation. Individual Market Portability Rules (Not Applicable to HIPAA Eligible Individuals). kff.org/other/state-indicator/individual-market-portability-rules/. Accessed July 21, 2014.

46. U.S. Preventive Services Task Force. Grade Definitions. www.uspreventiveservicestaskforce.org/uspstf/grades.htm. Accessed July 21, 2014.

47. The Henry J. Kaiser Family Foundation. How Do Medicaid Disproportionate Share Hospital (DSH) Payments Change under the ACA? kaiserfamilyfoundation.files.wordpress.com/2013/11/8513-how-do-medicaid-dsh-payments-change-under-the-aca.pdf. Accessed July 21, 2014.

48. Neuhausen K, Spivey M, et al. State Politics and the Fate of the Safety Net. *New England Journal of Medicine.* 2013(369):1675.

49. Mullin J. For States Not Expanding Medicaid, DSH Cuts Will Deal a Tough Blow. www.advisory.com/daily-briefing/blog/2013/09/for-states-not-expanding-medicaid-dsh-cuts-will-deal-a-tough-blow. Accessed July 21, 2014.

50. HealthCare.gov. Preventive Care Benefits. www.healthcare.gov/what-are-my-preventive-care-benefits/#part=1. Accessed July 21, 2014.

51. Centers for Medicare & Medicaid Services. Independence at Home Demonstration Fact Sheet. www.cms.gov/Medicare/Demonstration-Projects/DemoProjectsEvalRpts/downloads/IAH_FactSheet.pdf. Accessed July 21, 2014.

52. Ruggio M, Hurd P, et al. Summary of Anti-Fraud Provisions in the Affordable Care Act. www.leclairryan.com/files/Uploads/Documents/ACA%20Anti-Fraud%20Provisions%20slide%20deck%2008%2021%2013%20final.pdf. Accessed July 21, 2014.

53. Gold J. FAQ on ACOs: Accountable Care Organizations, Explained. www.kaiserhealthnews.org/stories/2011/january/13/aco-accountable-care-organization-faq.aspx. Accessed July 21, 2014.

54. Centers for Medicare & Medicaid Services. Shared Savings Program. www.cms.gov/Medicare/Medicare-Fee-for-Service-Payment/sharedsavingsprogram/index.html. Accessed July 21, 2014.

55. Centers for Medicare & Medicaid Services. Pioneer ACO Model. innovation.cms.gov/initiatives/Pioneer-ACO-Model/. Accessed July 21, 2014.

56. Medicare.gov. Costs in the Coverage Gap. www.medicare.gov/part-d/costs/coverage-gap/part-d-coverage-gap.html. Accessed July 14, 2014.

57. Smith S. ACA's Gradual Closure of Part D "Donut Hole" Saves $1,265 Per Beneficiary. health.wolterskluwerlb.com/2014/03/acas-gradual-closure-of-part-d-donut-hole-saves-1265-per-beneficiary/. Accessed July 21, 2014.

58. Wargo B. Everybody Just Relax! Medicare Isn't in Any Financial Trouble. completesenior.com/relax-medicare-financial-trouble/. Accessed July 21, 2014.

59. American Medical Association. Independent Payment Advisory Board. www.ama-assn.org/ama/pub/advocacy/topics/independent-payment-advisory-board.page. Accessed July 21, 2014.

60. Oberlander J, Morrison M. Failure to Launch? The Independent Payment Advisory Board's Uncertain Prospects. *New England Journal of Medicine.* 2013;369:105.

61. The Henry J. Kaiser Family Foundation. Status of State Action on the Medicaid Expansion Decision, 2014. kff.org/health-reform/state-indicator/state-activity-around-expanding-medicaid-under-the-affordable-care-act/. Accessed July 14, 2014.

62. Antos J. Medicaid Expansion under the ACA: Dollars and Sense? www.aei.org/outlook/health/entitlements/medicaid-chip/medicaid-expansion-under-the-aca-dollars-and-sense/. Accessed July 21, 2014.

63. The National Association of State Budget Officers. An Update of State Fiscal Conditions. www.nasbo.org/sites/default/files/NASBO%20Fall%202013%20Fiscal%20Survey%20of%20States.pdf. Accessed July 21, 2014.

64. Rick Scott: Medicaid Expansion Would Strain State Budgets. www.usnews.com/debate-club/is-medicaid-expansion-good-for-the-states/medicaid-expansion-would-strain-state-budgets. Accessed July 21, 2014.

65. Park E. CBO Finds Health Reform's Medicaid Expansion Is an Even Better Deal for States. www.cbpp.org/cms/index.cfm?fa=view&id=4131. Accessed July 21, 2014.

66. Medicaid.Alabama.gov. Medicaid Income Limits for 2014. medicaid.alabama.gov/documents/3.0_Apply/3.2_Qualifying_Medicaid/3.2_Medicaid_Income_Limits_Revised_2-7-14.pdf. Accessed July 21, 2014.

67. The Henry J. Kaiser Family Foundation. Where Are States Today? Medicaid and CHIP Eligibility Levels for Children and Non-Disabled Adults as of April 1, 2014. kff.org/medicaid/fact-sheet/where-are-states-today-medicaid-and-chip/. Accessed July 21, 2014.

68. The Henry J. Kaiser Family Foundation. The Coverage Gap: Uninsured Poor Adults in States That Do Not Expand Medicaid. kff.org/health-reform/issue-brief/the-coverage-gap-uninsured-poor-adults-in-states-that-do-not-expand-medicaid/. Accessed July 15, 2014.

69. The Henry J. Kaiser Family Foundation. Characteristics of Poor Uninsured Adults Who Fall into the Coverage Gap. kff.org/health-reform/issue-brief/characteristics-of-poor-uninsured-adults-who-fall-into-the-coverage-gap/. Accessed July 15, 2014.

70. Money Follows the Person. www.medicaid.gov/Medicaid-CHIP-Program-Information/By-Topics/Long-Term-Services-and-Supports/Balancing/Money-Follows-the-Person.html. Accessed July 21, 2014.

71. Kliff S. Obamacare Is About to Give Medicaid Docs a 73 Percent Raise. www.washingtonpost.com/blogs/wonkblog/wp/2012/12/21/obamacare-is-about-to-give-medicaid-docs-a-73-percent-raise/. Accessed July 21, 2014.

72. Centers for Medicare & Medicaid Services. New Loan Program Helps Create Customer-Driven Non-Profit Health Insurers. www.cms.gov/CCIIO/Resources/Grants/new-loan-program.html. Accessed July 21, 2014.

73. Selby J, Lipstein S. PCORI at 3 Years—Progress, Lessons, and Plans. *New England Journal of Medicine.* 2014;370:592.

74. Holtz-Eakin D, Ramlet MJ. Health Care Reform Is Likely to Widen Federal Budget Deficits, Not Reduce Them. *Health Affairs.* 2010;29(6):1136.

75. Congressional Budget Office. Updated Estimates of the Effects of the Insurance Coverage Provisions of the Affordable Care Act, April 2014. www.cbo.gov/sites/default/files/cbofiles/attachments/45231-ACA_Estimates.pdf. Accessed July 21, 2014.

76. Health Costs and History. Government Programs Always Exceed Their Spending Estimates. *Wall Street Journal.* Oct 20, 2009.

77. BlueCross BlueShield of North Carolina. In the Spotlight: ACA Taxes and Fees. www.bcbsnc.com/assets/hcr/pdfs/spotlight_taxes_and_fees.pdf. Accessed July 21, 2014.

78. Goldfarb Z, Somashekhar S. White House delays health-care rule that businesses provide insurance to workers. http://www.washingtonpost.com/politics/white-house-delays-health-care-rule-that-businesses-provide-insurance-to-workers/2013/07/02/f87e7892-e360-11e2-aef3-339619eab080_story.html. Accessed July 21, 2014.

79. Kliff S. Obamacare's Online SHOP Enrollment Delayed by One Year. www.washingtonpost.com/blogs/wonkblog/wp/2013/11/27/obamacares-online-exchange-for-small-businesses-is-delayed-by-one-year/. Accessed July 21, 2014.

80. Pear R. A Limit on Consumer Costs Is Delayed in Health Care Law. *The New York Times.* August 12, 2013.

81. Bagley N. The Legality of Delaying Key Elements of the ACA. *New England Journal of Medicine.* 2014(370):1967.

82. Mullaney T. Obama Adviser: Demand Overwhelmed Healthcare.Gov. *USA Today*; Oct 6, 2013.

83. Goldstein A. Obama administration will allow more time to enroll in health care on federal marketplace. www.washingtonpost.com/national/health-science/obama-administration-will-allow-more-time-to-enroll-in-health-care-on-federal-marketplace/2014/03/25/d0458338-b449-11e3-8cb6-284052554d74_story.html. Accessed July 21, 2014.

84. Budnick N. Cover Oregon: Health Exchange Failure Predicted, but Tech Watchdogs' Warnings Fell on Deaf Ears. *The Oregonian*. Jan 18, 2014.

85. Landler M, Shear M. Enrollments Exceed Obama's Target for Health Care Act. *The New York Times*. Apr 17, 2014.

86. Park H, Watkins D, et al. Health Exchange Enrollment Ended with a Surge. *The New York Times*. May 1, 2014.

87. Weaver C, Mathews A. Exchanges See Little Progress on Uninsured. *Wall Street Journal*. Jan 17, 2014.

88. Lopez G. Sorry, Republicans, Obamacare Enrollees Are Paying Their Bills. www.vox.com/2014/5/7/5690716/sorry-republicans-obamacare-enrollees-are-paying-their-bills. Accessed July 21, 2014.

89. Baker S. 15-20 Percent Aren't Paying Obamacare Premiums, Insurer Says. www.nationaljournal.com/health-care/15-20-percent-aren-t-paying-obamacare-premiums-insurer-says-20140402. Accessed July 21, 2014.

90. Long S, Kenney G, et al. Quicktake: Number of Uninsured Adults Falls by 5.4 million since 2013. hrms.urban.org/quicktakes/changeInUninsurance.html. Accessed July 21, 2014.

91. Sebelius K. Medicaid Enrollment Grows by More Than 3 million. www.hhs.gov/healthcare/facts/blog/2014/04/medicaid-chip-determinations-february.html. Accessed July 21, 2014.

92. Mangan D. President: 7.1 million Enrolled in Obamacare. www.cnbc.com/id/101543801. Accessed July 15, 2014.

93. McIntryre A. Forget the 7.1 Million: Obamacare's Real Enrollment Numbers Are Still to Come. theweek.com/article/index/259173/forget-the-71-million-obamacares-real-enrollment-numbers-are-still-to-come. Accessed July 21, 2014.

94. Sommers B. Number of Young Adults Gaining Insurance Due to the Affordable Care Act Now Tops 3 Million. aspe.hhs.gov/aspe/gaininginsurance/rb.cfm. Accessed July 21, 2014.

95. Mckinsey R: Only 14% of Obamacare Exchange Sign-Ups Are Previously Uninsured Enrollees. www.forbes.com/sites/theapothecary/2014/03/08/mckinsey-only-14-of-obamacare-exchange-sign-ups-are-previously-uninsured-enrollees/. Accessed July 21, 2014.

96. Roy A. Not Affordable Care Act: Opposing View. www.usatoday.com/story/opinion/2013/09/23/not-affordable-care-act-avik-roy-editorials-debates/2858175/. Accessed July 21, 2014.

97. Holtz-Eakin D, O'Neill J, et al. www.politico.com/static/PPM191_impact.html. Accessed July 21, 2014.

98. The Wall Street Journal. Obamacare's Plans Are Worse. online.wsj.com/news/articles/SB10001424052702303460004579192081764514664. Accessed July 21, 2014.

99. Owcharenko N. Mr. President, We Want Real Health Care Reform, Not Obamacare. dailysignal.com/2014/02/02/mr-president-want-real-health-care-reform-obamacare. Accessed July 21, 2014.

100. The National Review. The CBO's Obamacare Scorecard. www.nationalreview.com/article/370367/cbos-obamacare-scorecard-editors. Accessed July 21, 2014.

101. Balizet L. The Only Way Out. www.pnhp.org/news/2014/january/the-only-way-out. Accessed July 21, 2014.

102. The Patient Care Act. www.hatch.senate.gov/public/_cache/files/bf0c9823-29c7-4078-b8af-aa9a12213eca/The%20Patient%20CARE%20Act%20-%20LEGISLATIVE%20PROPOSAL.pdf. Accessed July 21, 2014.

103. Jost T. Beyond Repeal—a Republican Proposal for Health Care Reform. *New England Journal of Medicine*. 2014;320(10):894.

104. Gluck A. A Legal Victory for Insurance Exchanges. *New England Journal of Medicine.* 2014;370(10).

105. The Henry J. Kaiser Family Foundation. Kaiser Health Tracking Poll: March 2014. kff.org/health-reform/poll-finding/kaiser-health-tracking-poll-march-2014/. Accessed July 21, 2014.

106. The Henry J. Kaiser Family Foundation. Average Per Person Monthly Premiums in the Individual Market, 2010. kff.org/other/state-indicator/individual-premiums/. Accessed July 21, 2014.

107. McClellan M, McKethan AN, et al. A national strategy to put accountable care into practice. *Health Affairs.* 2010;29(5):982.

108. Sommers BD, Epstein AM. Why States Are So Miffed about Medicaid — Economics, Politics, and the "Woodwork Effect." *New England Journal of Medicine.* 2011;365(2):100-102.

109. Congressional Budget Office. The Budget and Economic Outlook: 2014 to 2024. www.cbo.gov/publication/45010. Accessed July 21, 2014.

110. Ander S, Newport F. After Exchanges Close, 5% of Americans Are Newly Insured. www.gallup.com/poll/171863/exchanges-close-americans-newly-insured.aspx. Accessed July 21, 2014.

Chapter 6
Health Care Providers
with Vikram Shankar

Health care is a huge industry in the U.S. It already accounts for more than one-tenth of all American workers and is projected to add more jobs than any other sector of the economy over the next 10 years,[1] especially with the passage of the Affordable Care Act (ACA) and subsequent influx of millions of newly insured patients into the health care system. The health care workforce can be quite complicated; if you walk into a hospital and start checking out work badges, you may end up being confused about who's who. What's a CNS? Is a DO the same as an MD? What does an LVN do? This chapter serves as a handy reference guide to the health care workforce—a quick snapshot of the many important professions who make health care happen.

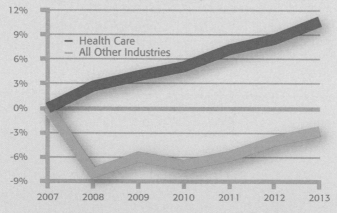

Percentage Job Change, 2007–2013

- Health Care
- All Other Industries

Joshua Wright, "Health Care's Unrivaled Job Gains and Where it Matters Most," Oct. 2013. Used with permission.

Training

Education

Educational requirements vary significantly for different health professions. Although some health care professionals receive all of their education on the job, the majority attend formal degree-granting programs that may last anywhere from nine months to 10 or more years.

Many health care providers complete doctoral degrees that are specific for each profession. Upon graduation, members of particular professions—physician assistants, podiatrists, and others—may enter postgraduate residency programs to receive additional training.

Licensing (i.e., Approval by the Government)

Licensing is legal approval from a state government to practice a profession. Licenses must be renewed every few years; usually, this requires a fee and completion of continuing education in the field. Only those who are licensed are allowed to use certain titles associated with each profession.

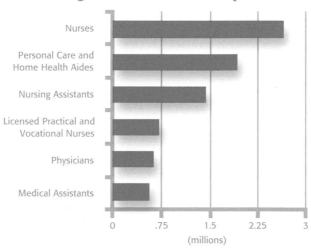

Largest Health Care Occupations

Bureau of Labor Statistics, "Occupational Employment and Wages," May 2013.

Certification *(i.e., Approval by a Professional Organization)*

Board certification is a formal recognition of competence from a nongovernmental, national professional organization. Two types of certification are common. For professions that are licensed, certification allows workers to demonstrate proficiency in specific practice areas (e.g., specialty physicians such as psychiatrists and cardiologists). For professions that aren't licensed, certification is a way of demonstrating quality to employers and the public. Some health care institutions require certification, even if the law does not.

Scope of Practice

In every state and for each licensed profession, laws regulate what health care providers can and cannot do. This is termed the "scope of practice," and it determines what diagnoses, treatments, and procedures a health care professional may perform in each state. Scope-of-practice regulations often differ significantly from state to state.

For example, although nurse practitioners (NPs) have the authority to prescribe medications in all 50 states, nearly every aspect of their authority varies across the country. Currently, 18 states[2] allow NPs to prescribe with complete autonomy, while the remaining states require some form of regulated physician oversight. In some states, NPs are only allowed to prescribe medications from a limited formulary set by the state. As you can see, this gets complicated very quickly.

Interprofessional Health Care Teams

Many newer models of health care delivery are organized around the concept of interprofessional, team-based medical care. Interprofessional care teams are composed of members from several different health professions who bring specialized knowledge, experience, and skills to the care of a given patient.[3]

Interprofessional health care teams are particularly effective in caring for patients with multiple, complex medical conditions such as diabetes, asthma, or cardiovascular disease. Let's consider the example of diabetes, which currently affects 8.3%[4] of the U.S. population and is expected to affect one-third of Americans by the year 2050. Diabetes and its related conditions can affect nearly every organ system, and optimal care must be coordinated among several health care providers—the physician who diagnoses the condition and prescribes treatment; the nurse who helps the patient learn how to take his or her medications and measure blood glucose properly; the physical therapist who works with activity limitations; the dietician who alters the patient's eating regimen; and the podiatrist who treats the patient's foot ulcers and other complications.[5] Pharmacists assist in selecting the proper medication regimens, and social workers can help ensure that the patient can afford—and remain adherent with—the medications prescribed. Leveraging the knowledge and skills of each health care provider ensures that treatment is focused on the patient's needs and results in improved health outcomes.

Interprofessional teams have long been a part of medical care in settings such as hospital ICUs and stroke care units. However, the team-based model has gradually been adopted in newer models of health care delivery such as Patient-Centered Medical Homes and Accountable Care Organizations.[6] The hope is that interprofessional care teams will improve the coordination and delivery of patient care while mitigating health care costs.[7] For example, new reimbursement models in the ACA based on shared savings or capitation could provide a revenue stream that can support non-physician team members through their potential impact on lowering costs. New payment and incentive structures emphasize developing such teams, but effective adoption and implementation of team-based care still faces significant challenges.

As far back as 1972, the Institute of Medicine (IOM) recognized that changing medical care to a team-based model would involve wholesale changes at several levels: organizational, administrative, instructional, and national. In particular, the IOM noted that academic health centers would need to introduce a more collaborative educational model among the various health professions, particularly through integrating classroom instruction and clinical education.[8] Furthermore, systemic "macro-level" factors such as governmental policies, reimbursement, and regulation—not to mention societal and cultural values regarding medical care—introduce even more complexity to this issue. A transformation to team-based care faces significant barriers, which will require both collaboration and creativity to overcome.[9]

Mid-level Providers

The Affordable Care Act is expected to introduce nearly 30 million newly insured Americans to the health care system beginning in 2014, which raises significant concerns about the ability of the U.S. health care workforce to meet this growing demand. This is especially relevant in light of the physician shortage, estimated to reach 91,500 by the year 2020.[10] Many experts contend that this provider shortage cannot be addressed simply through the growth of the physician workforce; rather, "mid-level providers" such as NPs (nurse practitioners) and PAs (physician assistants) must play significant roles within interprofessional health care teams in order to bridge this gap.[11]

Many experts suggest that expanding the roles of non-physician providers in patient care may help drive down health care costs, a primary goal of health care reform. For example, services provided by non-physician providers are reimbursed at lower rates by Medicare than identical services performed by physicians.[12] However, total spending may not be reduced because mid-level providers usually see fewer patients than physicians and may order more diagnostic testing.[13,14] Non-physician providers may also offer adaptability within the health care system because of their shorter training periods and ability to specialize in particular fields.[15]

Scope-of-Practice Reform

The roles and responsibilities of physicians and non-physician providers often overlap. For example, PAs and NPs can perform many of the primary care services typically provided by physicians, such as conducting physical exams, interpreting lab results, and counseling patients on preventive health measures.[16] Efforts to expand the roles of non-physician providers have increased scrutiny of scope-of-practice laws in each state, which specify the professional practice limits of health care providers.

Reform of scope-of-practice laws involves sensitive issues such as income, prestige, professional identity, and potential benefit or harm to patients. Notably, there has been some recent movement across state legislatures to ease practice restrictions for non-physician health care providers, particularly NPs and PAs. More than a dozen states now permit NPs to practice independently (without physician supervision),[2] and NPs can apply for full admitting privileges at many hospitals.[17] Similarly, a number of states permit nurse anesthetists to practice without physician supervision,[18] especially those with large rural populations and physician shortages. For example, more than 80% of Kansas hospitals providing surgical services rely solely on nurse anesthetists, rather than physicians, to provide anesthesia care.[19] Broadly, such legislative action has been supported by organizations such as the Institute of Medicine, which suggested that nurses "should practice to the full extent of their education and training" through the reform of state-level scope-of-practice laws.[20]

Although most agree that the spread of interprofessional health care teams has been a positive development, the move to allow some non-physician providers to practice in an independent, unsupervised setting is more controversial. Of note, several physician groups have expressed reservations about independent practice for these providers, contending that it would expand their responsibilities *beyond* their training. The American Academy of Family Physicians (AAFP) argues that NPs and PAs can serve important roles as part of physician-led care teams but are not substitutes for physicians themselves. Noting that physicians receive more than 20,000 total hours of medical training prior to practice independence—compared to between 2,800–5,350 hours for NPs—the AAFP argues that the "training and expertise [of a nurse practitioner] is not equal to that of a primary care physician."[21]

However, the American Association of Nurse Practitioners (AANP) suggests that "evidence supports [that] the quality of NP care is at least equivalent to that of physician care." In a position paper on nurse practitioner practice, the AANP contends that NPs can provide comparable levels of patient satisfaction and long-term care to that of physicians in primary care settings.[22] A small number of other studies have also shown that NPs can provide comparable health outcomes to primary care practices involving only physicians.[13,23-25] The Institute of Medicine writes, "No studies suggest that APRNs [advance practice nurses] are less able than physicians to deliver care that is safe, effective, and efficient or that care is better in states with more restrictive scope of practice regulations for APRNs. In fact, evidence shows that nurses provide quality care to patients, including preventing medication errors, reducing or eliminating infections, and easing the transition patients make from hospital to home."[26]

We should note, too, the preference of patients. A 2013 survey indicated that most patients prefer physicians to NP/PAs when selecting a new primary care physician, but that a majority of patients would opt to see an NP/PA "now" as opposed to waiting to see an MD for pressing conditions.[27]

Currently, as evidence regarding the safety and effectiveness of these non-physician providers in unsupervised practice is limited, this topic will continue to be vigorously debated. As the U.S. health care system evolves, so too will the roles, responsibilities, and scope of practice for non-physician practitioners. However, the diffusion of interprofessional team-based care and a growing health care provider gap will undoubtedly require the knowledge and skills of these non-physician providers, likely in a larger and more active role than they have had in the past.

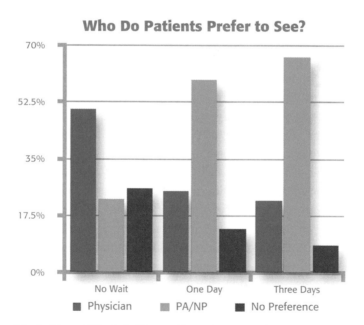

Who Do Patients Prefer to See?

Adapted from: Dill, et al., "Survey Shows Consumers Open to a Greater Role for Physician Assistants and Nurse Practitioners," June 2013. Note: Counts and percentages were weighted; see study for details. Scenarios were presented as follows: "Now imagine you have developed 1) a worsening cough or 2) frequent severe headaches over the past several weeks and decide that you need to seek medical care. You call the clinic and are told you can see a nurse practitioner or physician assistant today or tomorrow, or you can see a physician in 1 or 3 days. Which would you choose?"

Health Care Provider Reference Guide

This is a quick guide to the health care professionals you're most likely to come across. Each table includes the total number of persons in that profession, gender (when available), what they do, how they're educated, and more.

Assistant/Aide	NA/CNA/AA/CDA/PCT/many more
▸ Total number:	▸ 3.8 million[28]　　　　　Female: 89%　Male: 11%[29]
▸ Education:	▸ Some receive no formal training and learn on the job. Others attend 1-year certificate/diploma programs or 2-year associate's degree programs offered in technical and vocational schools, community and junior colleges, and universities.
▸ Licensing:	▸ State laws usually regulate scope of practice, but many states do not require a license for practice. National organizations are active in certification and continuing medical education.
▸ Average Salary:	▸ Varies based on role. Lowest and highest paid: • Nursing Aides: Hourly: $12.32; Annually: $25,620[28] • Occupational Therapy Aides: Hourly: $25.52; Annually: $53,090[28]
▸ Job Description:	▸ This category encompasses a wide variety of health care workers (excluding physician assistants and medical assistants) who are directed and supervised by licensed health care professionals. Aides are usually classified by the occupation of their supervisors: occupational therapy aides, anesthesia aides, etc. These workers perform a wide range of vital tasks in all health care settings. Contact with patients can be extensive or quite minimal, depending on specific job requirements.
	▸ The largest subtype, accounting for more than 40% of all aides and assistants, is nursing aides. Also known as orderlies or patient care technicians, nursing aides work under the supervision of registered nurses and practical nurses. They can perform many basic patient care duties, including helping patients eat, dress, and bathe; serving meals, making beds, and tidying up rooms; taking vital signs, helping patients ambulate, and escorting them to surgery or imaging. Nursing aides are also the primary caregivers in most nursing homes.

Audiologist	AuD
▸ Total number:	▸ 12,800[28] Female: 84% Male: 16%[30]
▸ Education:	▸ Typically attend 3–4-year programs, involving classroom, laboratory, and supervised clinical experiences. Coursework includes anatomy, physiology, and pathology of auditory and vestibular system, and focuses on evaluation and treatment of hearing and balance disorders.
▸ Licensing:	▸ Licensed in all 50 states, though some states require additional Hearing Aid Dispenser licenses.
▸ Average Salary:	▸ Hourly: $33.52; Annually: $69,720[28]
▸ Job Description:	▸ Audiologists work with patients who have hearing, balance, or other ear problems like tinnitus. They use a variety of tests to determine the severity and cause of hearing and balance disorders, and determine treatments on their own or in conjunction with the patient's medical team. Audiologists often fit and program hearing aids, middle ear implants, and cochlear implants; examine and clean ear canals; and provide rehabilitative strategies for patients with hearing loss. Many audiologists work for companies whose employees are at risk for noise-induced hearing loss, and others in schools where they administer auditory screening tests and rehabilitative and diagnostic services.

Health Care Chaplain/Hospital Chaplain	CC/BCC/CCC/BCCC
▸ Total number:	▸ 13,080,[28] many more volunteers
▸ Education:	▸ At least 100 hours of didactic and 300 hours of clinical training in a health care setting. Many health care chaplains also have Master of Divinity degrees or an equivalent.
▸ Licensing:	▸ Not state licensed. Several organizations offer voluntary board certification in clinical pastoral services, which requires a master's degree, clinical training, and supervised experience in a health care institution.
▸ Average Salary:	▸ Hourly: $23.37; Annually: $48,610[28]
▸ Job Description:	▸ Health care chaplains are responsible for attending to the spiritual needs of patients, especially in hospitals, nursing homes, and hospice services. Approximately 55% of hospitals employ chaplains, and religiously affiliated hospitals are more likely than secular hospitals to employ chaplains.[31] Chaplains may be trained clergy or lay people of any religion. Chaplains spend time one-on-one with patients, work with patients' families, provide spiritual support for medical staff, and may lead regular services in

(Continued) Health Care Chaplain/Hospital Chaplain	CC/BCC/CCC/BCCC

▸ Job Description: ▸ hospital chapels. In many hospitals, hospices, and long-term care facilities, chaplains are part of an interdisciplinary care team and are consulted to perform spiritual assessments and to determine a plan of care for the patient. Chaplains are often called to provide bereavement support for patients and their families in the last hours of life.

Chiropractor	DC

▸ Total number: ▸ 49,100[28]   Female: 19%   Male: 81%[29]

▸ Education: ▸ Typically complete a 4-year doctorate degree involving science classwork and supervised clinical rotations, with emphasis on musculoskeletal anatomy, spinal adjustment, manipulation, and radiology. Postgraduate training in 10 specialties[32] is available (orthopedics, acupuncture, etc.) but not required for practice.

▸ Licensing: ▸ Licensed in all 50 states.

▸ Average Salary: ▸ Hourly: $38.25; Annually: $79,550[28]

▸ Job Description: ▸ Chiropractors diagnose and treat patients with problems of the musculoskeletal system, especially back and neck pain. Many chiropractic treatments deal specifically with the spine, using manipulation of the spine as a primary intervention. Chiropractic medicine is based on the principle that spinal joint misalignments interfere with the nervous system and can result in lower resistance to disease and many conditions of diminished health.

▸ Chiropractors take the patient's health history; conduct physical, neurological, and orthopedic examinations; and may order laboratory tests. X-rays and other diagnostic images are important tools because of the chiropractic emphasis on the spine and its proper function. Chiropractors also analyze the patient's posture and spine using specialized techniques. For patients whose health problems can be traced to the musculoskeletal system, chiropractors manually adjust the spinal column.

▸ Some chiropractors use additional procedures in their practices, including heat, water, light, massage, ultrasound, electric currents, and acupuncture. They may apply supports such as straps, tape, braces, or shoe inserts. Chiropractors cannot prescribe drugs or perform major surgery.

Counselor

▸ Total number:	▸ 302,540[28]	Female: 69% Male: 31%[29]

▸ Education:
▸ Most complete an undergraduate degree before enrolling in a master's program in counseling, psychology, or social work.

▸ Licensing:
▸ All states require at least a master's degree, and voluntary national certification requires passing of a state-recognized exam through the National Board of Certified Counselors.

▸ Average Salary:
▸ Varies based on role, average annual wages are as follows: Substance abuse and behavioral disorder counselors: $41,090; Mental health counselors: $43,700; Rehabilitation counselors: $37,660[28]

▸ Job Description:
▸ Counselors help individuals, families, or groups cope with physical, mental, and emotional disorders. They perform a wide variety of tasks intended to support patients, and may be classified by their specific role.

▸ **Rehabilitation counselors** help people with disabilities resulting from birth defects, illness or disease, accidents, or other causes. They provide personal and vocational counseling; offer case management support; and arrange for medical care, vocational training, and job placement.

▸ **Mental health counselors** treat mental and emotional disorders and promote mental health. They are trained in a variety of therapeutic techniques to address issues such as depression, anxiety, substance addiction and abuse, suicidal impulses, stress, trauma, low self-esteem, and grief.

▸ **Substance abuse and behavioral disorder counselors** help people who have problems with alcohol, drugs, gambling, and eating disorders. Counseling can be done on an individual basis but is frequently done in a group setting and can include crisis counseling, daily or weekly counseling, or drop-in counseling supports.[33]

Dentist		DDS/DMD
▶ Total number:	▶ 155,700[28]	Female: 31% Male: 69%[29]
▶ Education:	▶ DDS programs last 4 years and require an undergraduate degree with specific science coursework. The first 2 years of dental school are primarily classroom-based, while the 3rd and 4th years are clinically based. Postgraduate training is not required, but around 20%[34] complete specialty training including orthodontics, oral and maxillofacial surgery (OMFS), etc. Some OMFS specialists complete 6-year joint dentistry/general surgery residencies and receive both an MD and a DDS upon graduation.	
▶ Licensing:	▶ Licensed in all 50 states.	
▶ Average Salary:	▶ Hourly: $78.48; Annually: $163,240[28]	
▶ Job Description:	▶ Dentists are the primary providers of tooth, gum, mouth, and masticatory system care in the U.S. They can perform many of the duties of physicians, including taking histories, ordering and interpreting imaging, making diagnoses, prescribing medication, and performing surgery, but are restricted to the oral cavity and masticatory system. Additional qualifications or training are required to carry out complex treatments such as dental implants and oral and maxillofacial surgery. Some dentists, especially dental surgeons, have full hospital privileges, while most others have courtesy privileges or no hospital relationships. The American Dental Association (ADA) recognizes 9 dental specialties, including pediatric dentistry, public health, and periodontics.[35]	

Dietician		RD/LD/LDN
▶ Total number:	▶ 59,530[28]	Female: 90% Male: 10%[29]
▶ Education:	▶ Two educational paths are possible at either the undergraduate or graduate level, and both involve science coursework including nutrition, chemistry, and physiology. Students can enter a coordinated program combining classroom instruction and clinical rotations, or can pursue a didactic classroom program followed by separate clinical rotations. Typically, 900 hours of clinical rotations are needed prior to taking the certification exam.	

201

(Continued) Dietician	RD/LD/LDN
▶ Licensing:	▶ Laws vary by state, but nearly half of registered dietitians are state-licensed.[36] The title "Registered Dietician" denotes graduation from an accredited dietetics program and passage of a national certification exam.
▶ Average Salary:	▶ Hourly: $27.00; Annually: $56,170[28]
▶ Job Description:	▶ Dietitians take detailed nutritional histories, assess metabolic and functional status, and work with other health professionals to develop appropriate diets for patients. This often involves designing diets to manage medical conditions like diabetes, or in response to treatments like chemotherapy. Dietitians are also centrally involved in selecting the feeding method (e.g., parenteral) and composition of nutritional support for patients who cannot eat, often as part of a multidisciplinary nutrition support team. RDs can specialize in areas such as pediatric or oncology nutrition.

Emergency Medical Technician/Paramedic	EMT
▶ Total number:	▶ 232,860 (excluding volunteers)[28] Female: 39% Male: 61%[29]
▶ Education:	▶ A high school diploma is typically required prior to entering a training program, and there are five levels of EMT training: First Responder, EMT-Basic (110 hours training), EMT-Intermediate/85, EMT-Intermediate/99 (200–400 hours), and EMT-Paramedic (1,000+ hours).[37,38] Paramedics are trained in anatomy and physiology as well as clinical skills such as advanced airway support and IV fluid management.[39]
▶ Licensing:	▶ Licensed in all 50 states, and most require certification by either the National Registry of EMTs or by state-specific programs.
▶ Average Salary:	▶ Hourly: $16.77; Annually: $34,870[28]
▶ Job Description:	▶ EMTs and paramedics are responsible for quickly responding to emergency situations, assessing and stabilizing victims' medical conditions, and transporting victims to the nearest medical facility via ambulance or helicopter. EMTs and paramedics operate in emergency medical services systems where a physician provides medical direction and oversight. Scope of practice depends on level of training and differs by state. Typical responsibilities also vary by training:

| *(Continued)* Emergency Medical Technician/Paramedic | EMT |

▸ Job Description:
- ▸ **EMT-Basic:** Noninvasive procedures such as bag-valve-mask ventilation, splinting, and automated external defibrillation.
- ▸ **EMT-Intermediate:** Starting IV lines, placing nasogastric tubes, and administering a limited number of medications, such as epinephrine and albuterol.
- ▸ **EMT-Paramedic:** Administering a greater number of medications orally or intravenously, including antipsychotics and narcotics; interpreting EKGs; endotracheal intubations; blood transfusions; and thoracic decompressions.[40]

Health Care Administrator

▸ Total number:
- ▸ 300,180[28]

▸ Education:
- ▸ Education varies greatly, with 52% holding a bachelor's degree, 31% a master's degree, and 10% having completed a post-bachelor's certificate program.[41] Some attend 2- or 3-year master's programs in health administration (MHA), public health (MPH), business administration (MBA), or public administration (MPA). Others are promoted health care practitioners like physicians or nurses with no formal management training.

▸ Licensing:
- ▸ All states require licensing for nursing home administrators, while licensing is generally not required for other areas of health care administration.

▸ Average Salary:
- ▸ Varies widely based on size of institution and administrative position, from $54,000/year for mid-level managers at outpatient/group practices to over $18 million/year[42] for CEOs of private insurance companies.

▸ Job Description:
- ▸ Health care administrators plan, direct, coordinate, and supervise the delivery of health care. These workers are either specialists in charge of specific clinical departments or generalists who manage entire facilities or systems. This broad category includes a wide range of workers, from CEOs of large health care networks to budgeting managers at small group practices. Some health care providers, especially those in solo practice, also perform administrative duties, but most health care institutions are operated by full-time health administrators. Some administrators, known as information managers, are responsible for the maintenance and security of all patient records. As electronic health records become more prevalent throughout the field, information managers will be crucial in building and maintaining these electronic systems.[43]

Home Health Aide/Personal Health Aide		HHA/PHA
▸ Total number:	▸ 1.9 million[28]	Female: 89% Male: 11%[29]
▸ Education:	▸ No specific education is required; most employers and states do not require a high school diploma. Aides are usually trained on the job. HHAs working for agencies reimbursed by Medicare or Medicaid must complete certain requirements, including courses on personal hygiene, safe transfer technique, infection control, and more. Overall, aides undergo 75 hours of training, including 16 hours of supervised practical experience and an examination.	
▸ Licensing:	▸ Voluntary certification available from the National Association for Home Care & Hospice, and some states require additional training in order to practice.	
▸ Average Salary:	▸ Hourly: $10.09; Annually: $20,990[28]	
▸ Job Description:	▸ Home health aides provide help to the disabled, chronically ill, elderly, cognitively impaired, and others who need assistance in their own homes or in residential facilities. They also assist people in hospices and day programs and help individuals with disabilities go to work and remain engaged in their communities. Aides provide light housekeeping and homemaking tasks such as laundry, changing bed linens, shopping for food, planning and preparing meals. Aides also may help clients get out of bed, bathe, dress, and groom. Some accompany clients to doctors' appointments or on other errands. Aides may go to the same home every day or week for months or even years and often visit four or five clients on the same day.	

Medical Assistant		MA/CMA/RMA/CCMA/NCMA
▸ Total number:	▸ 571,690[28]	Female: 94% Male: 6%[29]
▸ Education:	▸ Some attend 1-year certificate/diploma programs or 2-year associate's degree programs, but education varies greatly. Programs are available in high schools, technical and vocational schools, community and junior colleges, and universities. Overall, 65% of medical assistants have completed a post-high school certificate program, 18% hold an associate's degree, and 10% hold only a high school diploma.[41]	
▸ Licensing:	▸ No state requires licensing, but some require permits for certain procedures such as phlebotomies and injections. Voluntary certification programs and examinations are available from national organizations.	
▸ Average Salary:	▸ Hourly: $14.80; Annually: $30,780[28]	

(Continued) Medical Assistant — MA/CMA/RMA/CCMA/NCMA

▶ Job Description:
▶ Medical assistants are jack-of-all-trades helpers for physicians and other health care providers. They perform administrative and clinical duties to keep offices running smoothly and to ensure patients are cared for. Specific tasks vary widely by place of employment, but common responsibilities include taking vital signs; preparing and maintaining examination and treatment areas; preparing patients for examination; assisting with procedures and treatments; preparing and administering medications; recognizing, screening, and following up on patient test results; collecting and processing patient specimens for medical tests; scheduling appointments; claims submission; and monitoring third party reimbursement.[44] Many medical assistants advance to other professions in the health care field such as medical administration or nursing.

Medical Coder — CPC/CCS/RHIT

▶ Total number:
▶ 182,370[28]

▶ Education:
▶ Some receive no formal training and learn on job, while others attend 6-month or 1-year certificate/diploma programs or 2-year associate's degree programs. Training programs are available in high schools, technical and vocational schools, and community and junior colleges. Overall, 48% have earned a high school diploma, and 20% hold an associate's degree.[45]

▶ Licensing:
▶ Coders are not licensed by any state. Several organizations offer voluntary national certification.

▶ Average Salary:
▶ Hourly: $17.68; Annually: $36,770[28]

▶ Job Description:
▶ Medical coders specialize in codifying patients' medical information for reimbursement purposes. They assign a code to each diagnosis and procedure using classification systems software. The classification system determines the amount for which health care providers will be reimbursed if the patient is covered by Medicare, Medicaid, or other insurance programs using the system. Coders may use several coding systems, such as those required for ambulatory settings, physician offices, and long-term care.

Medical Scientist	
▸ Total number:	▸ 104,280[28] Female: 52% Male: 48%[29]
▸ Education:	▸ Although there are no specific educational requirements to be a medical scientist, most have a PhD in an area of biological science. PhD programs last 3–6 years and are university-based, involving a combination of science classwork and independent research. Prior to graduation, students must compile and present dissertations of original research, and may then enter postdoctoral apprenticeships that last 1–3 years in laboratories of accomplished scientists. Students may also enter 8–9 year programs housed in medical schools that lead to both an MD and a PhD degree.
▸ Licensing:	▸ Although medical scientists are not licensed by any state, those who interact medically with patients or administer drugs must be licensed physicians (MD or DO).
▸ Average Salary:	▸ Hourly: $43.38; Annually: $90,230[28]
▸ Job Description:	▸ Medical scientists conduct biomedical research to advance knowledge of life processes and of other living organisms that affect human health, including viruses, bacteria, and other infectious agents. They also engage in laboratory research, clinical investigation, technical writing, drug development, regulatory review, and related activities. For example, medical scientists involved in cancer research may formulate a combination of drugs that will mitigate the effects of the disease. They can then work with physicians to administer these drugs to patients in clinical trials, monitor their reactions, and observe the results. In addition to developing treatments for medical conditions, medical scientists attempt to discover ways to prevent health problems. For example, they may study the link between smoking and lung cancer or between alcoholism and liver disease. Many medical scientists divide their time between clinical practice and research activities.

Nurse		RN
▸ Total number:	▸ 2.7 million[28]	Female: 90% Male: 10%[29]
▸ Education:	▸ Several educational paths available to become an RN:	
	▸ Bachelor's Degree (BSN): 3- to 4-year university program. Time may be split between university and nursing college or completed at one institution	
	▸ Accelerated BSN: 12- to 18-month program for students with non-nursing bachelor's degrees; leads to a BSN at a university or nursing college	
	▸ Associate's Degree (ASN, AAS, ADN): 2-year program at community or junior college	
	▸ Diploma: 3-year program at hospital-based school of nursing or community college	
	▸ Master's entry level (MN, MSN, CNL): 3- to 4-year graduate program for students with non-nursing bachelor's degrees	
	▸ Completion of one of these paths allows a graduate nurse to take the national licensure exam. Master's programs are also available for RNs who wish to become advanced practice nurses or nurse educators. Overall, 45% of nurses hold a bachelor's degree, 38% hold an associate's degree, 10% hold a master's degree, and 7% earn a diploma.[46] Around 15% of RNs complete advanced education and certification in one of more than 70 specialties.[47]	
▸ Licensing:	▸ Licensed in all 50 states.	
▸ Average Salary:	▸ Hourly: $32.66; Annually: $67,930[28]	
▸ Job Description:	▸ Nurses are the largest group of employees in the health care field, and they often spend more time with the patient and family members than any other health care professional. RNs play a variety of roles in both inpatient and outpatient institutions, and their work responsibilities vary accordingly. We examine this profession in greater detail on the following pages.	

PROFESSIONAL RESPONSIBILITIES

Every new patient admitted to a hospital undergoes an initial nursing assessment by an RN to determine the patient's physical condition and functional status. During the course of a patient's stay, nurses conduct ongoing assessments, identify patient problems, maintain a plan of care, perform interventions, and evaluate the results of interventions within their scope of practice. Such independent interventions include symptom management, patient and family education, skin and wound care, and grief counseling. Other actions are specified by institutional protocol or in the "patient orders" that are submitted by physicians and other health care providers. Because nurses spend the most time with patients, they often confer with other members of the care team regarding the management of patients.

RNs are responsible for a broad range of patient care activities, including vital sign monitoring; starting, regulating, and maintaining IVs and catheters; delivering oxygen therapies, medication administration; obtaining blood and tissue specimens for laboratory testing; ambulating patients; educating patients and their family members; supervising and directing practical nurses and nursing aides; discharge planning and instruction; and charting and maintaining the medical record.

In most hospitals, nurses are assigned to a care team in a single location or medical unit. A "clinical nurse manager" is the RN responsible for administration and supervision of that unit; when the nurse manager is off duty, another RN acts as a "charge nurse," supervising the other RNs and patients and conferring with the medical staff. All hospitals employ a Chief Nursing Executive (title may differ by institution) to provide central nursing administration.

ADVANCED NURSING PROFESSIONS

Advanced practice nurses (APRN) are RNs who have completed specialized graduate training and have a broader scope of practice for diagnosis and treatment than do RNs. There are four types: clinical nurse specialists, nurse anesthetists, nurse midwives, and nurse practitioners. The U.S. has more than 200,000 practicing APRNs.[28] All four types are licensed separately in all 50 states.

RNs who wish to become an advanced practice nurse must complete a master's program (MSN). Most programs are two years and require a BSN and RN license for admission. Most programs require clinical work experience as an RN in a related field before applying. Many schools also offer post-master's clinical doctorate (DNP) programs lasting two to three years. These graduates often use their doctoral education to become experts in a specialized field like diabetes or pediatrics, while others go on to health care administration. Nursing research doctorate programs (DNS/DNSc) are also available, lasting four to six years, for nurses who would like to focus on research as a primary career.

APRN (Advanced Practice Nurse) Specialties

Nurse Practitioners (NP/CNP/CRNP) can perform most of the duties of physicians, such as taking histories, making diagnoses, prescribing medication and performing limited procedures. In many states, they must be supervised or have a collaborative practice agreement with physicians; such supervision may range from consultations after each patient encounter to meetings every few months. About one-fifth of NPs have hospital admitting privileges.[48] NPs are allowed to prescribe medications in all 50 states, but some states also require the co-signature of a physician and/or restrict the prescription of controlled substances. Average yearly salary is $95,070.[28]

Clinical Nurse Midwives (CNM/CNMW/CM/NM /CPM) are providers of OB/GYN services with an emphasis on pregnancy and childbirth. Their scope of practice is similar to that of NPs and PAs; they can diagnose and treat most conditions in the OB/GYN field, but in most states must have a professional relationship with a physician. CNMs can also treat male partners for STDs and provide medical care for the normal newborn for the first month of life. They are legally allowed to write prescriptions in some states but not others. Average yearly salary is $92,230.[28]

Clinical Nurse Specialists (CNS) have a similar education and scope of practice as NPs but with a different focus. Whereas NPs treat individual patients with a variety of conditions, CNSs usually focus on a single condition or specialty, such as oncology or critical care, for which they provide advanced nursing care. In addition to direct patient care, CNSs engage in teaching, mentoring, research, management, and systems improvement.[49] CNSs are allowed to prescribe medications in some states.[50]

Nurse Anesthetists (CRNA/NA) specialize in administering sedation and anesthesia. Scope of practice varies by state; some require physician relationships, but 17 states allow CRNAs to practice without physician supervision. NAs are the primary provider of anesthesia in many rural locations. Unique in nursing, more than 40% of NAs are male.[51] Average yearly salary is $157,690.[28]

Practical Nurse/Vocational Nurse		LPN/LVN
▸ Total number:	▸ 705,200[28]	Female: 92% Male: 8%[29]
▸ Education:	▸ Programs usually require a high school diploma and are 12–18 months with a focus on practical clinical education. These programs are offered in high schools, technical and vocational schools, hospitals, community and junior colleges, and universities.	
▸ Licensing:	▸ Licensed in all 50 states.	
▸ Average Salary:	▸ Hourly: $20.39; Annually: $42,200[28]	
▸ Job Description:	▸ Practical nurses provide patient care under direction of an RN or physician. They perform many of the same duties as RNs but are not allowed to make diagnoses or perform certain procedures and functions (specifics vary from state to state). For example, they may be allowed to remove catheters and IV lines but not place them. Major functions of LPNs in the hospital include administering medications; taking and recording vital signs; dressing wounds; feeding patients; assisting patients with dressing, hygiene, bathroom care, and walking; monitoring inputs and outputs; and taking EKGs. In the outpatient setting, LPNs may also be responsible for making appointments and other clerical duties in the physician's office, or for assisting patients with activities of daily living, if employed in nursing homes or in home health care. Often, LPNs are charged with directing and supervising nursing aides and other support personnel. Many LPNs go on to become RNs at a later date.	

Occupational Therapist		OT/OTR/MOT/MSOT/OTD
▸ Total number:	▸ 108,800[28]	Female: 88% Male: 12%[29]
▸ Education:	▸ Master's programs (MSOT/MOT) are graduate degrees designed to prepare generalist practitioners. These last 2.5 years and include both classroom instruction and 6 months of supervised clinical experience. Coursework includes anatomy, applied neuroscience, physiology, and psychology. Doctoral programs (OTD) last 3.5 years and focus on concentrated areas of practice expertise such as neurorehabilitation or pediatrics or professional role specializations including research, education, or management.	
▸ Licensing:	▸ Licensed in all 50 states.	

(Continued) Occupational Therapist	OT/OTR/MOT/MSOT/OTD
▸ Average Salary:	▸ Hourly: $36.73; Annually: $76,400[28]
▸ Job Description:	▸ Occupational therapists help people with medical conditions and disabilities achieve greater function and independence in their lives by promoting meaningful activities or "occupations." Occupations include activities of daily living such as dressing, cooking, eating, working, and going to school. The goal of occupational therapy is to improve patients' performance and participation in everyday life activities, thereby improving well-being.
	▸ Exercises may be used to increase strength and dexterity to restore function after illness or injury, while compensatory or alternative strategies may be taught for coping with permanent disabilities. For example, OTs select and teach the use of adaptive devices like wheelchairs, orthoses, eating aids, and dressing aids. OTs teach cognitive-behavioral or self-management strategies to promote client-centered care and long-term quality of life for those living with chronic health conditions. Therapists also may collaborate with patients and employers to modify home or work environments so that patients can function more independently.
	▸ Hospital-based OTs are often centrally involved in the discharge planning process, along with nurses, case managers, and physical therapists. The OT assesses the patient in order to recommend the appropriate level of care for the patient post-discharge—e.g., nursing home, rehab, home with assistance, etc.

Optometrist		OD
▸ Total number:	▸ 32,040[28]	Female: 39% Male: 61%[52]
▸ Education:	▸ Typically, 3–4 years of undergraduate work are required before admission to a 4-year doctoral program of optometry. The first 2 years consist of classroom and laboratory work, followed by 2 years of supervised clinical rotations. Residency is not required, but around 20% complete specialty training (pediatrics, contact lens fitting, etc.).[53]	
▸ Licensing:	▸ Licensed in all 50 states.	
▸ Average Salary:	▸ Hourly: $52.80; Annually: $109,810[28]	

(Continued) **Optometrist**		**OD**
▸ Job Description:	▸	Optometrists are the primary providers of eye care in the U.S. They can perform many of the duties of physicians, including taking histories, ordering and interpreting imaging, and diagnosing conditions of the eye, but are restricted from performing surgery in all but a handful of states. Optometrists can prescribe medication in most states but may be barred from prescribing controlled substances. Optometrists are commonly confused with other eye health professionals; to clarify, ophthalmologists are physicians who specialize in eye care, whereas opticians make, fit, and help patients select eye glasses and contacts.

Pharmacist		**PharmD/RPh/BS Pharmacy**
▸ Total number:	▸	286,400[28] Female: 56% Male: 44%[29]
▸ Education:	▸	At least 2 years of undergraduate work are required before admission to 4-year programs, although many programs combine undergraduate and graduate work into a 6-year degree. Classroom learning is combined with laboratory instruction and supervised clinical rotations. 15% complete 1–2 year postgraduate residencies in general, clinical, or specialty pharmacy practice;[54] residency is increasingly required to work in clinical settings.
▸ Licensing:	▸	Licensed in all 50 states.
▸ Average Salary:	▸	Hourly: $56.09; Annually: $116,670[28]
▸ Job Description:	▸	Pharmacists are responsible for receiving prescriptions and preparing medicines for patients. They are also legally responsible for educating patients about medications and work with physicians to optimize pharmacotherapy, for example by reducing dangerous drug interactions and side effects. Pharmacists that work in hospitals or other institutions as part of health care teams may also be consulted by physicians and asked to help select medications or design medication regimens for inpatient treatment. In many states, pharmacists enter into "collaborative practice agreements" with physicians, which may enable them to modify medication regimens and prescribe a limited number of drugs. Pharmacists can administer medications and immunizations, although this varies from state to state. Pharmacists' scope of practice is much greater in federal settings such as the VA.

Physical Therapist	PT/DPT/MPT/MSPT/BSPT
▸ Total number:	▸ 204,200[28] Female: 61% Male: 39%[29]
▸ Education:	▸ The most common degree for physical therapy is the clinical doctorate (DPT), obtained after 3 years of graduate studies. The curriculum involves supervised clinical rotations and science classwork in subjects including anatomy, physiology, exercise physiology, and biomechanics, among others. Postgraduate residency programs focus on patient care in a defined area of practice such as orthopedics, and require a minimum of 1,500 hours of training within a period of 9–36 months.
▸ Licensing:	▸ Licensed in all 50 states.
▸ Average Salary:	▸ Hourly: $38.39; Annually: $79,860[28]
▸ Job Description:	▸ Physical therapists have unique expertise in diagnosis and treatment of movement-related conditions that limit strength, balance, coordination, flexibility, and functional independence. Common conditions they treat include musculoskeletal injuries such as sprains, chronic pain, broken bones, arthritis, and amputations. They may also work with patients with neurological disorders such as stroke, multiple sclerosis, and cerebral palsy.
	▸ Treatments employed by PTs may include therapeutic exercises, stretching, range-of-motion exercises and mobilization, functional training, manual therapy, use of assistive and adaptive devices/equipment to enhance function, and therapeutic modalities and electrical stimulation to manage pain. They often prescribe long-term exercise plans for patients to complete on their own following treatment; these exercises are intended to improve functional independence, prevent further symptoms from developing, and promote neuromusculoskeletal health. About 7% of PTs are board certified in one of eight specialties, including sports and women's health.[55]
	▸ Physical therapists are often confused with physiatrists (also known as PM&Rs), who are physicians who specialize in physical rehabilitation. PTs and physiatrists often work together in caring for patients with musculoskeletal injury.

Physician	MD (Allopathic)/DO (Osteopathic)
▸ Total number:	▸ 623,380[28] (93% MD/7% DO)[56] Female: 36% Male: 64%[29]
▸ Education:	▸ MD programs require an undergraduate degree and last 4 years. The first 2 years of medical school are pre-clinical and classroom based, and coursework includes anatomy, physiology, pharmacology, pathology, and more. Years 3 and 4 are clinically based, and students work as part of care team in hospitals and clinics. Rotations during these years include internal medicine, surgery, psychiatry, pediatrics, and others.
	▸ DO programs are very similar to MD programs in length, structure, and content with a few key differences. Osteopathic medical education places a strong emphasis on primary care. Students also receive training in osteopathic manipulative treatment, a hands-on treatment where DOs use their hands to diagnosis and treat patients.
▸ Licensing:	▸ Licensed in all 50 states.
▸ Average Salary:[57]	▸ Varies based on specialty: 37% of physicians work in primary care, 63% in specialties[63]: • Primary Care: Hourly: $60.65; Annually: $149,053[a] • Internal Med/Pediatric Subspecialties: Hourly: $84.85; Annually: $235,815; • Surgery: Hourly: $92.10; Annually: $260,830
▸ Job Description:	▸ Physicians diagnose and treat injury and disease and are the primary educators and advisers of patients. Physicians examine patients; obtain medical histories; and order, perform, and interpret diagnostic tests. They prescribe medications and perform surgeries and other procedures. Physician specialties include anesthesiology, family medicine, internal medicine, pediatrics, obstetrics and gynecology, psychiatry, and surgery, as well as many others. Although only one-fifth of health expenditures go directly to physician services, their clinical decisions determine up to 90% of total health expenditures.[64]
	▸ Osteopathic physicians have the same scope of practice as allopathic physicians. DOs are more likely to practice in rural or underserved communities than MDs, and are also more likely to pursue careers in primary care. Other than that, their practices are virtually indistinguishable, and DOs and MDs often work together.

a   These salaries are drawn from a 2008 study of hourly wages for physicians; highest was neurosurgery at $132/hour. A 2014 Medscape physician survey found the highest annual salary was orthopedics at $413,000/year and lowest was infectious diseases at $174,000/year.

GRADUATE MEDICAL EDUCATION

Physicians' degrees are awarded after completion of four years of medical school, but graduates must complete postgraduate residency training[b] in a medical specialty before they're allowed to practice medicine. During residency, these new physicians see and treat patients under the supervision of more experienced physicians. Residency programs are generally hospital-based, and are governed by the Accreditation Council for Graduate Medical Education (ACGME).[58] The National Resident Matching Program uses an algorithm to match students with residencies based on mutual preference; those students who enter "the match" are obligated to accept their given positions. Specialties include well-known fields such as internal medicine, general surgery, pediatrics, and anesthesiology and smaller disciplines such as medical genetics and nuclear medicine. Residency lasts from three years (family medicine, pediatrics, etc.) to six or more years (neurosurgery), and training can further be extended with sub-specialty fellowships.

Salaries reflect that residents are trainees: Residents don't have to pay tuition, but their wages (around $50,000 yearly) are more like educational stipends than physicians' incomes. These wages come mostly from Medicare and Medicaid funds,[59] the limited nature of which also determines the number of residency slots. The Balanced Budget Act of 1997 placed a limit on the number of Medicare-supported resident slots, meaning that there has been a steady cap on the number of residents. This has obvious implications for the number of physicians, as discussed in Chapter 1. The Affordable Care Act (ACA) doesn't change this cap, although it does redistribute some funds to promote primary care.

A number of other health care professions—including pharmacy, optometry, and dentistry—also offer postgraduate residencies, but these residencies aren't required for practice.

---

b   Think "Scrubs" and "Grey's Anatomy" without the glamour.

Physician Assistant · PA/RPA/LPA

▸ Total number:	▸ 86,700[28] · Female: 65% Male: 35%[29]
▸ Education:	▸ Training programs are 2–3 years after completion of an undergraduate degree and include clinical training in several areas along with instruction in anatomy, physiology, clinical medicine, ethics, and more. Most programs grant master's degrees, while others grant bachelor's or associate's degrees, or certificates. Postgraduate residency is not required but available for specialization in a field (e.g., surgery, emergency medicine).
▸ Licensing:	▸ Licensed in all 50 states.
▸ Average Salary:	▸ Hourly: $45.36; Annually: $94,350[28]
▸ Job Description:	▸ Physician assistants can perform most of the duties of a physician, such as taking histories, making diagnoses, prescribing medication, and performing limited procedures, but they must do so under physician supervision. Supervision can vary from direct observation by the physician to daily meetings between the PA and physician. However, in some rural or inner-city clinics, physicians may only be present for one or two days per week, and PAs act as the principal care providers for most patients. Surgical PAs assist surgeons during procedures and suture wounds but do not perform surgery themselves. PAs are allowed to prescribe medications in all 50 states, but some states also require the co-signature of a physician or restrict the prescription of controlled substances.

Podiatrist · DPM

▸ Total number:	▸ 8,850[28]
▸ Education:	▸ At least 90 hours of undergraduate study are necessary before admission to a college of podiatric medicine. Programs last 4 years, with 2 years of classroom and laboratory work and 2 years of supervised clinical rotations. After graduation, podiatrists complete a 3-year residency similar to that of physicians.
▸ Licensing:	▸ Licensed in all 50 states.
▸ Average Salary:	▸ Hourly: $64.94; Annually: $135,070[28]
▸ Job Description:	▸ Podiatrists are the primary providers of foot and ankle care in the U.S.[60] They can perform many of the duties of physicians, including taking histories, ordering and interpreting imaging, making diagnosis, prescribing medication, and performing surgery, but their work is restricted to the foot and ankle. Hospital relationships vary by institution; some podiatrists are granted full hospital admitting privileges, and some co-admit with physicians. Many podiatrists specialize in areas such as sports medicine or pediatrics.

Clinical Psychologist	CP/LCP/LP/PsyD
▸ Total number:	▸ 104,480[28]　　　　　　Female: 58%　Male: 42%[61]
▸ Education:	▸ A bachelor's degree is required before entering graduate-level programs. Programs last 4–5 years and include classroom education, original research, and writing and presenting a dissertation. Graduates entering clinical careers enter a "match," similar to that of physicians, which places them in 1-year clinical internships across the country.
▸ Licensing:	▸ Licensed in all 50 states. In most states, licensure requires a doctoral degree in psychology, 1 year of postdoctoral fellowship, a dissertation, supervised clinical experience, and completion of a certification exam.
▸ Average Salary:	▸ Hourly: $34.96; Annually: $72,710[28]
▸ Job Description:	▸ Clinical psychologists are mental health providers that focus on the mind and behavior. They assess and diagnose mental illnesses such as mood, anxiety, behavior, and adjustment disorders, and treat these conditions through interactive therapy. Common interventions include cognitive restructuring, behavioral management strategies, motivational interviewing, and modifying family patterns of interaction. Some psychologists complete advanced training to become board-certified in a specialty. Health psychologists are a specialty of clinical psychologists that often work in health care settings. Their activities include identifying strategies to promote adherence and increase coping, making behavioral changes to support physical and emotional health, and helping with pain management.

Social Worker	LSW/LICSW/LCSW/CSW/LCS/LMSW

▸ Total number: ▸ 273,920[28]   Female: 80%   Male: 20%[29]

▸ Education: ▸ Both undergraduate and graduate programs exist for social work. Bachelor's degree programs at universities or colleges last 3–4 years, with a curriculum that includes both classwork and 400 hours of supervised clinical experience. Coursework includes social work values and ethics, human behavior, social research methods, and more. Master's degree programs require an undergraduate degree, but not necessarily in social work; these programs last 2 years and include a minimum of 900 hours of supervised field instruction.

▸ Licensing: ▸ Many states offer a tiered system of social work licenses based on education and clinical experience (e.g., Social Worker, Clinical Social Worker, and Independent Clinical Social Worker).

▸ Average Salary: ▸ Hourly: $21.78; Annually: $45,300[28]

▸ Job Description: ▸ Social workers in hospitals and other medical settings are often responsible for helping patients with non-medical issues that nevertheless affect their health. For example, many hospital-based social workers make discharge plans for patients to ensure that they will go to a safe place to recuperate upon leaving the hospital. This may include finding shelter for homeless patients, arranging home health care services, transferring patients to rehabilitation centers, and planning for follow-up visits at the hospital or clinic. Social workers often help indigent patients apply for health insurance and financial support and manage advance directives, patient support groups, and patient transportation.

▸ Social workers are found in a number of other health care roles, including therapist; in fact, clinical social workers working as therapists are the nation's largest group of mental health service providers.[62] They are employed in a variety of settings, including outpatient clinics, substance abuse rehabilitation centers, employee assistance programs, and private practice. Social workers focus on mental health problems in the context of a patient's overall lifestyle and will often work to change lifestyle or living conditions to alleviate mental problems. Services may include individual and group therapy, outreach, crisis intervention, social rehabilitation, and teaching skills needed for everyday living. Many social workers work outside the medical field; they are not included here.

Speech–Language Pathologist — SLP

▸ Total number:	▸ 125,050[28] Female: 96% Male: 4%[30]
▸ Education:	▸ Undergraduate coursework in communication sciences is prerequisite for graduate speech pathology training. Programs are 2–3 years and include classroom instruction and supervised clinical rotations. Coursework includes normal and abnormal function of communication and swallowing organs and systems.
▸ Licensing:	▸ Voluntary certification is offered by American Speech-Language-Hearing Association and includes a national examination that satisfies most state licensing requirements.
▸ Average Salary:	▸ Hourly: $35.56; Annually: $73,790[28]
▸ Job Description:	▸ Speech–language pathologists work with patients who have impairments in speaking, producing, or comprehending language, and with cognition and swallowing that result from congenital or acquired disease, syndrome, or injury. SLPs help patients develop or recover functional communication and swallowing skills.
	▸ For individuals with little or no speech capability, speech–language pathologists may select augmentative or alternative communication methods, including automated devices and sign language, and teach their use. They teach patients how to make sounds, improve their voices, or improve their oral or written language skills to communicate more effectively. They also teach individuals how to strengthen muscles or use compensatory strategies to swallow without choking or inhaling food or liquid.

Technician/Technologist — XT/RDMS/CPhT/NMT/CVT/more

▸ Total number:	▸ 2.6 million[28] Female: 81% Male: 19%[29]
▸ Education:	▸ Many technicians receive no formal training and learn on the job. Others attend 6 month–1 year certificate/diploma programs, 2-year associate's degree programs, or 4-year bachelor's degree programs, which are offered in technical and vocational schools, community and junior colleges, and universities.
▸ Licensing:	▸ Many states do not require licensing. Voluntary certification is offered by national organizations after completing continuing education and passing standardized exams.

(Continued) Technician/Technologist	XT/RDMS/CPhT/NMT/CVT/more
▸ Average Salary:	▸ Varies based on role. Lowest and highest paid: • Ophthalmic technicians: Hourly: $17.44; Annually: $36,280[28] • Nuclear medicine technicians: Hourly: $34.60; Annually: $71,970[28]
▸ Job Description:	▸ This category encompasses a wide variety of health care workers (excluding EMTs) who deal primarily with specialized medical equipment. Examples include sonographers, who operate ultrasounds; pharmacy technicians, who prepare medicines; and radiology technologists, who operate imaging equipment like CT or MRI scanners. Specific responsibilities vary by title and institution. Generally, a health care professional such as a physician will order a test or treatment for a patient; technicians and technologists are then responsible for using their equipment to complete the order in a timely and accurate manner. Technicians and technologists work under the broad supervision of a physician but most of their day-to-day activities are performed independently.

References

1. Bureau of Labor Statistics. Health Care: BLS Spotlight on Statistics. www.bls.gov/spotlight/2009/health_care/. Accessed July 11, 2014.
2. The Henry J. Kaiser Family Foundation. Nurse Practitioner Prescribing Authority and Physician Supervision Requirements for Diagnosis and Treatment. kff.org/other/state-indicator/nurse-practitioner-autonomy/. Accessed July 11, 2014.
3. Greiner AC, Knebel E. *Health Professions Education: A Bridge to Quality.* Committee on the Health Professions Education Summit.
4. Centers for Disease Control and Prevention. 2011 National Diabetes Fact Sheet. www.cdc.gov/diabetes/pubs/factsheet11.htm. Accessed July 11, 2014.
5. Hellquist K, Bradley R, et al. Collaborative Practice Benefits Patients: An Examination of Interprofessional Approaches to Diabetes Care. *Health and Professional Practice.* 2012;1(2).
6. American College of Physicians. ACP: Patient-Centered Medical Home Overview. www.acponline.org/running_practice/delivery_and_payment_models/pcmh/understanding/index.html. Accessed July 11, 2014.
7. Iglehart JK. A New Day Dawns for Workforce Redesign. *Health Affairs.* 2013;32(11):1870.
8. National Center for Interprofessional Practice and Education. Iom 1972 Report: "Educating for the Health Team." nexusipe.org/resource-exchange/iom-1972-report-educating-health-team. Accessed July 15, 2014.

9. Interprofessional Education Collaborative Expert Panel. Core Competencies for Interprofessional Collaborative Practice. www.aacn.nche.edu/education-resources/ipecreport.pdf. Accessed July 15, 2014.

10. Association of American Medical Colleges. Physician Shortages to Worsen without Increases in Residency Training. www.aamc.org/download/153160/data/physician_shortages_to_worsen_without_increases_in_residency_tr.pdf. Accessed July 14, 2014.

11. Dower C, Moore J, et al. It Is Time to Restructure Health Professions Scope-of-Practice Regulations to Remove Barriers to Care. *Health Affairs.* 2013;32(11):1971.

12. Cunningham R. On Workforce Policy, Consensus Is Hard to Find. *Health Affairs.* 2013;32(11):1871.

13. Laurant M, Reeves D, et al. Substitution of Doctors by Nurses in Primary Care. *Cochrane Database of Systematic Reviews.* 2005(2).

14. Hemani A, Rastegar D, et al. A Comparison of Resource Utilization in Nurse Practitioners and Physicians. www.acponline.org/clinical_information/journals_publications/ecp/novdec99/hemani.htm. Accessed July 14, 2014.

15. Bodenheimer TS, Smith MD. Primary Care: Proposed Solutions to the Physician Shortage without Training More Physicians. *Health Affairs.* 2013;32(11):1881.

16. American Academy of Physician Assistants. What Is a PA? www.aapa.org/landingquestion.aspx?id=290. Accessed July 14, 2014.

17. Taylor B. Nurse Practitioner Takes on Pivotal Role at Critical Access Hospital. www.chausa.org/publications/catholic-health-world/article/march-1-2014/nurse-practitioner-takes-on-pivotal-role-at-critical-access-hospital. Accessed July 15, 2014.

18. American Association of Nurse Anesthetists. Federal Supervision Rule/Opt-out Information. www.aana.com/advocacy/stategovernmentaffairs/Pages/Federal-Supervision-Rule-Opt-Out-Information.aspx. Accessed July 14, 2014.

19. Kansas Association of Nurse Anesthetists. Kansas CRNA Practice. www.kana.org/information/crnapractice/. Accessed July 15,2014.

20. Institute of Medicine of the National Academies. *The Future of Nursing: Leading Change, Advancing Health.* 2010.

21. American Academy of Family Physicians. Scope of Practice Kit: What Is a Physician? www.aafp.org/dam/AAFP/documents/advocacy/workforce/scope/Restricted/ES-statescopeofpracticekit-051513.pdf. Accessed July 14, 2014.

22. American Association of Nurse Practitioners. Quality of Nurse Practitioner Practice. www.aanp.org/images/documents/publications/qualityofpractice.pdf. Accessed July 14, 2014.

23. Naylor MD, Kurtzman ET. The Role of Nurse Practitioners in Reinventing Primary Care. *Health Affairs.* 2010;29(5):893.

24. Horrocks S, Anderson E, et al. Systematic Review of Whether Nurse Practitioners Working in Primary Care Can Provide Equivalent Care to Doctors. *BMJ.* Apr 6 2002;324(7341):819.

25. Everett C, Thorpe C, et al. Physician Assistants and Nurse Practitioners Perform Effective Roles on Teams Caring for Medicare Patients with Diabetes. *Health Affairs.* 2013-11-01 2013;32(11):1942.

26. Institute of Medicine of the National Academies. The Future of Nursing: Focus on Scope of Practice. www.iom.edu/Reports/2010/The-Future-of-Nursing-Leading-Change-Advancing-Health/Report-Brief-Scope-of-Practice.aspx?page=2. Accessed July 14, 2014.

27. Dill MJ, Pankow S, et al. Survey Shows Consumers Open to a Greater Role for Physician Assistants and Nurse Practitioners. *Health Affairs.* Jun 2013;32(6):1135.

28. Bureau of Labor Statistics. Occupational Employment Statistics. www.bls.gov/oes/home.htm. Accessed May 12 2014.

29. Bureau of Labor Statistics. Current Population Survey. www.bls.gov/cps/cpsaat11.pdf. Accessed July 21, 2014.

30. American Speech-Language-Hearing Association. Highlights and Trends: Member and Affiliate Counts, Year-End 2013. www.asha.org/uploadedFiles/2013-Member-Counts-Year-End-Highlights.pdf. Accessed July 15, 2014.

31. Cadge W, Freese J, et al. The Provision of Hospital Chaplaincy in the United States: A National Overview. *South Med J.* Jun 2008;101(6):626.

32. Shaw G. Chiropractic Specialties on the Rise. www.acatoday.org/content_css.cfm?CID=2323. Accessed July 14, 2014.

33. Bureau of Labor Statistics. What Mental Health Counselors and Marriage and Family Therapists Do. www.bls.gov/ooh/community-and-social-service/mental-health-counselors-and-marriage-and-family-therapists.htm#tab-2. Accessed July 14, 2014.

34. American Dental Education Association. After Dental School. www.adea.org/dental_education_pathways/Pages/AfterDentalSchool.aspx. Accessed July 14, 2014.

35. American Dental Education Association. Dental Practice: Survey of Dental Practice Series. dev.ada.org/1619.aspx. Accessed July 14, 2014.

36. Rogers D. Compensation and Benefits Survey 2013: Education and Job Responsibility Key to Increased Compensation. *Journal of the Academy of Nutrition and Dietetics.* 2014;114(1):17.

37. National Registry of Emergency Medical Technicians. EMT-Basic Re-Registration. web.archive.org/web/20071028093612/nremt.org/EMTServices/rr_basic_history.asp. Accessed July 15, 2014.

38. National Registry of Emergency Medical Technicians. EMT-Intermediate/99. www.nremt.org/nremt/about/reg_int99_history.asp. Accessed July 14, 2014.

39. Lauro J, Sullivan F, et al. Emergency medical technician education and training. *Rhode Island Medical Journal.* 2013; 96(12):31.

40. Wisconsin Department of Health Services. Wisconsin EMS Scope of Practice. www.dhs.wisconsin.gov/ems/License_certification/scope_of_practice.htm. Accessed July 14, 2014.

41. O*NET Online. Summary Report for Medical and Health Services Managers. www.onetonline.org/link/summary/11-9111.00#Education. Accessed July 15, 2014.

42. Wagner N. The Money Pit: Health Insurance Executives' Pay. www.thedoctorwillseeyounow.com/content/healthcare/art2914.html?getPage=1. Accessed July 15, 2014.

43. Bureau of Labor Statistics. Occupational Outlook Handbook. www.bls.gov/ooh/healthcare/medical-records-and-health-information-technicians.htm#tab-6. Accessed July 15, 2014.

44. Tache S CS. Medical Assistants in California. www.futurehealth.ucsf.edu/Content/29/2004-05_Medical_Assistants_in_California.pdf. Accessed July 14, 2014.

45. O*NET Online. Medical Records and Health Information Technicians. www.onetonline.org/link/summary/29-2071.00#Education. Accessed July 14, 2014.

46. National Center for Health Workforce Analysis. The U.S. Nursing Workforce: Trends in Supply and Education. bhpr.hrsa.gov/healthworkforce/reports/nursingworkforce/nursingworkforcefullreport.pdf. Accessed June 28, 2014.

47. Ridge R. Nursing Certification as a Workforce Strategy. *Nursing management.* 2008;39(8):50.

48. Sipe TA, Fullerton JT, et al. Demographic Profiles of Certified Nurse-Midwives, Certified Registered Nurse Anesthetists, and Nurse Practitioners: Reflections on Implications for Uniform Education and Regulation. *Journal of Professional Nursing.* 2009;25(3):178.

49. American Association of Colleges of Nursing. AACN Statement of Support for Clinical Nurse Specialists. www.aacn.nche.edu/publications/position/CNS.pdf. Accessed July 14, 2014.

50. National Council of State Boards of Nursing. APRN Maps. www.ncsbn.org/2567.htm. Accessed July 14, 2014.

51. American Association of Nurse Anesthetists. Certified Registered Nurse Anesthetists at a Glance. www.aana.com/ceandeducation/becomeacrna/Pages/Nurse-Anesthetists-at-a-Glance.aspx. Accessed July 14, 2014.

52. American Optometric Association. Practicing Optometrists and Their Patients. www.aoa.org/Documents/optometrists/2012_Practicing_ODs-Executive_Summary.pdf. Accessed July 14, 2014.

53. American Optometric Association. Residency Program Opportunities. www.aoa.org/optometrists/for-educators/classroom-tools/residency-program-opportunities?sso=y. Accessed July 14, 2014.

54. Knapp KK, Shah BM, et al. Visions for Required Postgraduate Year 1 Residency Training by 2020: A Comparison of Actual Versus Projected Expansion. *Pharmacotherapy.* 2009;29(9):1030.

55. American Board of Physical Therapy Specialties. ABPTS Certified Specialists Statistics. www.abpts.org/About/Statistics/. Accessed July 15, 2014.

56. Association of American Medical Colleges. 2012 Physician Specialty Data Book. https://www.aamc.org/download/313228/data/2012physicianspecialtydatabook.pdf. Accessed July 15, 2014.

57. Leigh JP, Tancredi D, et al. Physician Wages across Specialties: Informing the Physician Reimbursement Debate. *Arch Intern Med.* Oct 25 2010;170(19):1728.

58. American Association of Colleges of Osteopathic Medicine. Allopathic and Osteopathic Medical Communities Commit to a Single Graduate Medical Education Accreditation System. www.acgme.org/acgmeweb/portals/0/PDFS/Nasca-Community/SingleAccreditationRelease2-26.pdf. Accessed July 14, 2014.

59. Dower C. Health Policy Brief: Graduate Medical Education. *Health Affairs.* 2012.

60. Illinois Podiatric Medical Association. Podiatry Facts & Statistics. ipma.net/displaycommon.cfm?an=1&subarticlenbr=15. Accessed July 14, 2014.

61. Michalski D, Mulvey T, et al. 2008 APA Survey of Psychology Health Service Providers. www.apa.org/workforce/publications/08-hsp/. Accessed July 21, 2014.

62. American Board of Examiners in Clinical Social Work. Clinical Supervision: A Practice Specialty of Clinical Social Work. www.abecsw.org/images/ABESUPERV2205ed406.pdf. Accessed July 14, 2014.

63. Health Resources and Services Administration. The Physician Workforce: Projections and Research into Current Issues Affecting Supply and Demand. http://bhpr.hrsa.gov/healthworkforce/reports/physwfissues.pdf. Accessed Apr 12, 2011.

64. Eisenberg J. Physician utilization: the state of research about physicians' practice patterns. *Medical Care.* 2002;40(11):1016.

Suggested Reading

Health care is an exciting and rapidly changing field, and our book only scratches the surface. For those of you who would like to learn more, we've listed some supremely useful books, journals, and websites below. Many others are listed on our website at **HealthCareHandbook.com/SuggestedReading.** Hope you enjoy!

On the Internet

RAND Health [rand.org/health], The Commonwealth Fund [commonwealthfund. org/publications/], and Robert Wood Johnson Foundation [rwjf.org/en/research-publications/research-features/] *These three nonprofit organizations produce some of the best reports and original research on the health care system that you can find anywhere. Extra kudos to RWJF's DataHub, a user-friendly health statistics visualization tool.*

Kaiser Family Foundation [kff.org] *If we could force you to go to this website, we would. This is an incredible resource, chock-full of information, well-explained, and free. It may be Elisabeth's favorite thing in the world.*

Kaiser Health News [kaiserhealthnews.org] *Phenomenal source for high-quality health care news on a wide swath of topics.*

The Incidental Economist [theincidentaleconomist.com] *A fantastic blog that's regularly updated with crucial insights and analysis of health economics and health policy. Make sure to check out their "Healthcare Triage" series on YouTube.*

The Health Care Blog [thehealthcareblog.com] *Includes submissions from physicians, economists, PhDs, and pundits on a huge range of topics across the political spectrum.*

Sarah Kliff [vox.com/authors/sarah-kliff] *One of the best (and most prolific) health care reporters working today. Does a great job of simplifying complex topics.*

Data.gov [data.gov/health] *The biggest repository of health care data out there; includes everything from infection rates at different hospitals to Medicare spending records to records of baby names in New York.*

TIME Magazine's "Bitter Pill" [time.com/198/bitter-pill-why-medical-bills-are-killing-us] *This amazing article details the movement of money in the health care system—who's making it, who's spending it, and why. Highly recommended.*

Capybara Madness [gianthamster.com/] *Has nothing to do with health care but does showcase the capybara, the world's most amazing animal.*

"Sick Around the World" from PBS Frontline [pbs.org/wgbh/pages/frontline/sickaroundtheworld/]: *This documentary compares and contrasts the health care systems of several first-world nations. It's the easiest way to get up to speed on the major types of health systems and how they work. Plus, the video is only 30 minutes.*

Journals

Health Affairs [healthaffairs.org] *The premier journal for health service research and policy commentary.*

New England Journal of Medicine [nejm.org], collections in "Health Policy and Reform" and "Medicine and Society," and Journal of the American Medical Association [jama.com], collections in "Health Care Delivery," "Health Care Reform," and "Health Policy/Health Economics": *America's two leading medical journals also feature some of the most important research and opinion pieces in health policy and delivery. We've listed the relevant collections for you here.*

Books

Health Care Delivery in the United States by Anthony Kovner, et al., and *Delivering Health Care in America*, by Leiyu Shi and Douglas Singh: *These lengthy tomes provide the most comprehensive and in-depth information about the U.S. health care system.*

Understanding Health Policy, by Thomas Bodenheimer and Kevin Grumbach: *More accessible and less textbookish than the preceding two; this book focuses much more on the policy side of health care.*

Crisis of Abundance: Rethinking How We Pay for Healthcare, by Arnold Kling: *Written by a libertarian economist, this book proposes a specific reform plan and highlights the trade-offs that must be dealt with in any health care system.*

The Social Transformation of American Medicine and *Remedy and Reaction*, by Paul Starr: *Social Transformation is the definitive history of health care in the U.S., and will give you a much better understanding of how we got where we are today. Remedy and Reaction details the history of American health care reform, including the ACA.*

The Immortal Life of Henrietta Lacks, by Rebecca Skloot: *Gripping account of a medical research breakthrough that provides an entirely different perspective on the scientific world and how it affects patients.*

Overtreated, by Shannon Brownlee: *Highlights the significant geographic variation in health care in the U.S. and how that variation can lead to unnecessary treatment.*

Mama Might Be Better Off Dead, by Laurie Kaye Abraham: *Follows a poor family with a host of medical and financial problems for a year in 1989. Though some of the obstacles presented are now outdated, a surprising number are not. Provides an excellent view into what it's like to be sick and on Medicaid.*

The Gold Standard: The Challenge of Evidence-Based Medicine, by Stefan Timmermans and Marc Berg: *The gold standard itself of EBM scholarship.*

Index

About the Authors

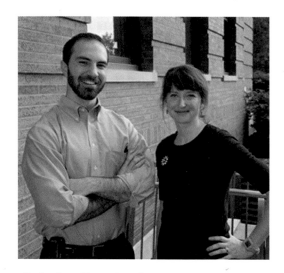

Elisabeth Askin and Nathan Moore are graduates
of the MD program at the Washington University
School of Medicine in St. Louis, Missouri. Elisabeth
is a resident physician in Internal Medicine at the
University of California-San Francisco, and Nathan is
a resident physician in Internal Medicine at Barnes-
Jewish Hospital/Washington University in St. Louis.
They both graduated from the University of Texas
at Austin and took time off after graduating. They
met in medical school and bonded over how much
they miss breakfast tacos.